The Reiki Beginner's Bible

How to Increase Your Energy, Restore Your Health and Feel Amazing Every Day

Copyright © 2015 by Tai Morello

Table of Contents

Introduction - A Brief History of Reiki 1

Chapter 1 - What is Reiki? 7

Chapter 2 - The Five Principles of Reiki 14

Chapter 3 - The Importance of Initiation 19

Chapter 4 – Choosing the Right Practitioner 20

Chapter 5 – How to Receive Reiki Attunements 24

Chapter 6 - The 7 Chakras 29

Chapter 7 - Reiki Level 1 33

Chapter 8 - Reiki Level 2 36

Chapter 9 - The Three Pillars of Reiki 38

Chapter 10 – Introduction to Alternative Reiki Healing Systems 41

Chapter 11 - Level I Self-Healing Techniques 45

Chapter 12: Level I Healing Techniques for Others 55

Chapter 13: Level II Self Healing Techniques 61

Chapter 14 : Level II Healing Techniques for Others 62

Chapter 15 - Healing Relationships 65

Chapter 16 - Transforming Negative Situations and Problems 68

Chapter 17 - Aura Cleansing Exercises 70

Chapter 18 - How to Increase Your Life Force Energy 72

Chapter 19 - Using the Power of Reiki to Attract anything you want 74

Chapter 20 - The Importance of Diet and Exercise 76

Chapter 21: Meditation for Exploring Your Connection to Reiki..... 78

Chapter 22 - Reiki for Animals, Children and the Elderly 86

Chapter 23 - Reiki and Other Healing Modalities 89

Chapter 24 – Reiki Healing Tools for Practitioners 90

Chapter 25 – Detecting and Healing Negative Energy: Techniques and Meditation 95

Conclusion - Tips to Maintain a Daily Practice............................. 100

Introduction - A Brief History of Reiki

While many of the world's great religions and spiritual paths talk about hands-on (or "laying of hands") healing, the art and science of energy healing had been mostly lost to the western world. Recently, there has been a resurgence of interest and practice in energy healing work, due in part to the holistic and alternative health movement's gaining significantly momentum from social media, documentaries, and public figures (such as celebrities, scientists, nutritionists, and even politicians) championing the transformative impact on their lives and the lives of others. The most popular method of energy healing to date is Reiki. Roughly translated as "guided spirit" in Japanese, Reiki is universal, life-force energy that is present in all things, across all times, spaces, and places. Reiki, essentially, is the essence of our physical, spiritual, emotional, and psychic world and operates according to the quantifiable laws and principals shared by physics, thermodynamics, and biofeedback. To receive or give Reiki is to augment this naturally occurring life-force energy to reset and strengthen its natural flow throughout the body, spirit, and energetic planes in order to sustain health and vitality. Reiki accelerates, liberates, and enhances all naturally occurring healing processes that our bodies unique employ simply because it interacts with the direct source, cause, processes and principals that lend to well-being, balance, and homeostasis. Reiki requires that we acknowledge our interconnectedness to the collective of energy in and outside of our bodies, and, that this collective must flow harmoniously otherwise its stagnancy will culminate in dis-ease (physical, emotional, and even spiritual).

Traditionally, those interested in receiving or giving Reiki are instructed to learn its rich origin history and lineage from the East to the West. This history is typically honored in its traditional oral format for Reiki students, in honor of the founder's (Dr. Mikao Usui) desire to teach as many people as possible. His format, the Usui Reiki Ryoho Hikkei (translating to "Usui's Reiki Healing Handbook"), is known universally today as "Usui Reiki". Usui Reiki is comprised of several key mindsets for embodying Reiki practice, the symbols required to attune oneself or another to interact with Reiki, how to teach Reiki to oneself and others, and the several sacred hand positions for self- and other-healing.

Dr. Mikao Usui, a Buddhist monk from Japan, "discovered" Reiki in the late 1800s in Japan. Dr. Usui, hailing from a family of doctors and devout Buddhists, was passionate about integrating medicine, theories of energy, and religious practice to create an integrated and inclusive energy healing system. Usui was specifically devoted to figuring out how an energy healing system could exist and sustain itself without borrowing or depleting energy from oneself or another source. If such an system could be created or discovered, Usui believed, then it would be more accessible, inviting, and powerful for individuals to not only be open to learning and using it, but also creating a larger community of healers. According to various sources, Dr. Usui, who dabbled in many different professions throughout his life, was once working as a college teacher. One of his students came up to him and asked him how Jesus had performed the many miracles talked about in the Bible. Dr. Usui became deeply intrigued by the question and he set out on a mission to find the answer. During one of Usui's intensive trainings and studies, he was called to attend Isyu Guo (a 21 day long experience that required him to live in a cave on Mount Kurama, fast, and pray in solitude). During his last day, Usui had a vivid and enlightened vision of sacred symbols drawn into the rocks of the mountainside. These symbols became the Usui Reiki symbols necessary to not only attune oneself and another to give Reiki, but also to give Reiki.

Upon the conclusion of his time at Mount Kurama, Dr. Usui moved to the large city of Kyoto, where he set up his school and healing clinic for Reiki. It was in Kyoto that Dr. Usui came to find the perfect hand placements for healing oneself and others, as well as the creation of the key tenants for mindfully practicing and embodying Reiki in one's life (also known as the Gainen or "Reiki Principles"). Dr. Usui started practicing Reiki on himself and the people close to him. After achieving great success through the practice, in 1922, Dr. Usui decided to open a training hall in Aoyama, Harajuku, Tokyo. Soon Dr. Usui's fame and popularity spread like wildfire. People traveled from far and wide to receive healing from him and to learn the art of Reiki healing. While in traditional Japanese society, healing arts were usually closely guarded as a family secret, Dr. Usui decided to empower the general public with the ability to heal through the power of Reiki.

In his debut handbook that he released ("Usui Reiki Ryoho Hikkei"), Dr. Usui talked about his intentions of making the method freely available to the world. He was against the idea of only a select few people possessing this healing power. He envisioned a better and healthier world, wherein, everyone would be able to experience the grace of the Divine. Dr. Usui's Reiki center was incredibly popular for these progressive ideas and leadership. Dr. Usui's methods for teaching his students (also known as "Shoden" or "beginner students") included the following: attunement to Reiki energy through a full-day ceremony, meditation, recitation of the Gainen/Reiki Principles, healing hand positions, and specialized curriculum and hand positions for treating specific illnesses, ailments, and accute mental disorders. Dr. Usui also instated two additional, powerful teaching treatises: 'Secret Method to Invite Happiness' and 'Miraculous Medicine to Cure All Diseases'.

In September 1923, a catastrophic earthquake hit Japan's Kanto district. There was massive destruction everywhere with many people left homeless and injured. Dr. Usui asked some of his students to extend a helping hand as a gesture of unconditional love. Due to the charitable work that Dr. Usui and his students did, his fame and popularity grew even more. Around the year 1925, Dr. Usui was visited by a party of naval officers at his teaching and healing center in Kyoto. In this group, there was also Chujiro Hayashi, who is the accredited as the second most important figure in the history and evolution of Reiki practice and history. Hayashi was so moved and impressed with the power of Reiki that he resigned from his former position as a naval officer and became a devout student of Dr. Usui's. During his study, Hayashi transferred his knowledge and experience as a naval officer and medic and exclusively pursued study on developing new hand positions for treating and preventing specific diseases, illnesses, injuries, and chronic conditions. Hayashi's vision and personal quest as a Reiki practitioner was to disseminate it so far across Japan that its use would be universal and as second-nature as self-prescribing medicine or going to the doctor. As such, he was entirely devoted to exploring how Reiki could cure, prevent, or treat any ailment or illness known in existence. Hayashi's commitment to the relationship between Reiki and illness manifested the third most important figure in Reiki (and is responsible for its existence in the West via the United States): Mrs. Hawayo Takata.

Mrs. Hawayo Takata was an Hawaiian-American woman of Japanese descent. After the passing away of her sister and husband, her health took a serious downturn. She traveled to Japan in order to find a doctor who could perform an operation that was deemed critical for restoring her health. While in Japan, she tried exploring other healing modalities and finally found herself in the clinic of Chujiro Hayashi.

With regular practice, Mrs. Takata's health improved dramatically over a relatively short period of time. She was amazed by the results and requested Chujiro Hayashi to teach her how to initiate others into the practice. Takata was a revered student of Hayashi; and so, while on his deathbed, he assigned Takata a mission to aggressively disseminate and share the teachings and practice as far and wide as possible. At this time, Japan was in turmoil from World War II and Takata took it upon herself to "save the world" by not only preserving the teachings of Reiki but taking it across the Pacific to the United States. After about a year, Mrs. Takata returned back to Hawaii and set up her own clinic. Unlike Usui and Hayashi, Taka never recorded her personal approach to Reiki and disseminated her knowledge via classes and verbal instruction alone. Takata is accredited for developing the two Level system of Reiki: 1 and 2. Reiki Level 1 focuses on the self and other. Level 1 Reiki students and practitioners are provided with attunement for Reiki and the hand positions. Reiki Level 2 focuses on how energy acts across time and space and enables students to heal events, timelines, prayers, and emotional energy as well as send Reiki to another person, place, or thing that is not occupying the same physical space or in physical proximity to the practitioner. Level 2 Reiki students receive additional attunements and are also trained in the three symbols that enable them to send Reiki across multiple dimensional planes in space, time and place in order to conduct distance healings. Later on, she not only initiated many into Level 1 and 2 Reiki but also made more than 20 Reiki masters. It was through the work of these masters that Reiki spread all over the world. When considering learning or receiving Reiki, it is imperative to ensure that the practitioner's lineage is directly descended and traceable to at least Takata, for she holds the direct teachings from Dr. Usui and Hayashi.

Simultaneously, Reiki became extremely popular with the officers of the armed forces as it does not require any equipment and can be done anywhere. Thanks to his rapidly growing popularity, Dr. Usui kept receiving requests to teach in many different cities. He graciously accepted these requests and traveled to the cities of Hiroshima, Kure, Sage and later on, Fukuyama. It was in Fukuyama that Dr. Usui died of a stroke at the age of 60.

Dr. Usui's memorial stone introduces him as a man who studied many different religions. His liberal attitude led him to adopt a mission to help build a better world and teach everyone who wanted to learn the art of Reiki healing. His memorial is one of the most frequently visited spots in Kyoto for disciples of Reiki all around the globe.

Current practitioners of Reiki all across the globe, therefore, owe their legacy to Mrs. Hawayo Takata and her teacher, Chujiro Hayashi. Without their work and passionate dedication to making energy healing accessible to all persons outside of Japan, Reiki would have likely remained unknown to the western world.

Chapter 1 - What is Reiki?

The word 'Reiki' has been formed with the root 'rei' meaning Higher Power or Divine Wisdom and 'ki' meaning life force energy. Reiki is, therefore, a flow of grace that heals the entire person. A session of Reiki involves sending life force energy to all the key energy centers in the body. This removes blockages which are considered to be the root cause of all diseases.

Reiki brings about powerful positive results in not just physical diseases but also in the case of mental and emotional problems. A typical session of Reiki feels deeply relaxing and rejuvenating. All Reiki practitioners and receivers of Reiki energy report feeling a sense of deep inner peace and calmness.

Dr. Usui describes Reiki as "something absolutely original and cannot be compared with any other spiritual path in the world ... This is why I would like to make this method freely available to the public for the well-being of humanity. Each of us has the potential of being given a gift by the divine, which results in the body and soul becoming unified. In this way, with Reiki, a great many people will experience the blessing of the divine .. our Reiki is an original therapy, which is build upon the spiritual power of the universe."

Ms. Takata, a later disciple of the Usui Reiki practice, in her interviews and teachings describes Reiki as belonging from a larger entity, stating: "I believe there exists One Supreme Being – the Absolute Infinite – a Dynamic Force that governs the world and universe. It is an unseen spiritual power that vibrates and all other powers fade into insignificance beside it. So, therefore, it is Absolute! This power is unfathomable, immeasurable, and being a universal life force, it is incomprehensible to man ... I shall call it, 'Reiki' because I studied under that expression ... Reiki ... comes from the Great Spirit, the Infinite!"

For individuals facing a physical, mental or emotional health issue, no matter how minor or severe, Reiki helps the body and spirit to accelerate its natural processes for healing and stability. As a result, these health issues are either significantly shortened, require less aggressive means of external healing (i.e. surgery or medication), have reduced or more mild symptoms, and, in some cases, completely vanish altogether. No matter how dire the health challenge, Reiki elevates our dire and ability to live and persevere by alleviating symptoms, reducing pain, easing our emotional anxiety and distress, and even peacefully accept and welcome death.

The Reiki healing experience is entirely guided by Reiki and Reiki alone. That is, the healer (whether it is you or another person), is not actively channeling this force into their hands, spirits, or even in your body: they are simply calling the existing Reiki to strengthen itself and use the sacred hand positions to assist Reiki's orientation into the proper energy points throughout the human body. Reiki is not a part of any religion or spiritual tradition: it is simply a tool, like massage, that enables our bodies to re-align and heal itself. To practice Reiki is to be in and of service to the miraculous and powerful abilities that energy can do for good. As a result, many Reiki Masters and students apply Reiki outside of the healing arena and use Reiki to support the positive development of political and social events, personal life, spirituality and religious traditions, and across environments.

BECOMING A STUDENT OF REIKI

The commitment to learning Reiki for oneself or to heal others is a life-long relationship to energy and the responsibility of healing. Those interested in becoming Reiki practitioners or students of Reiki undergo the following process:

- Identifying an Usui Reiki Master to attune them. Reiki Masters can be found at a variety of healing, wellness, and spiritual centers. When the student is really ready, the Master does indeed, show up. Prospective students often meet their Masters through change or in a transitory period of needing deep healing for themselves.

- Participating in a 1-2 full day ceremony that includes the following: receiving the attunements to have Reiki sealed in your hands and body for life, learning the history of Reiki, learning and meditating to the principles of Reiki, learning and practing the self-healing hand positions, learning and practicing the hand positions necessary for healing others, and incorporating Reiki throughout their lives as a practice and mindset.

- The 21 Day Period and Healing Crisis. This is specialized pledge for students that lasts over the course of 21 days. Students will physiologically, emotionally, and mentally feel the transformative effects of receiving the Reiki attunements through miraculous and sudden healings (that may also manifest themselves as illness, stress, or synchronistic events).

THE 21 DAY PERIOD

Upon initiation, every student takes a pledge to continue the practice for at least 21 days. The number 21 is considered to hold an important significance across many different religions and spiritual paths. Even Christianity recommends fasting and praying for a period of 21 days as a necessity for spiritual growth.

In the practice of Reiki, the student experiences a deep inner transformation and healing during the 21 day period. Upon initiation, a lot of hidden traumas and health issues might come to the surface. It is similar to homeopathy in this respect as the problems might come to the surface in full force. However, one must not get discouraged as these issues are coming up to be resolved and released completely. If, instead of getting overwhelmed, the student continues his practice with grit and determination for the 21 day period, then his life is guaranteed to change.

Talking about my own experience, when I was little, I suffered from severe nyctophobia which is an irrational and extreme fear of the night. I couldn't bear being alone and every time I would find myself alone in the dark, my heart would beat so hard that I would feel as if it is going to bounce out of my chest. I can't recall how many times I lied awake in bed simply staring at the ceiling completely covered in sweat and my heart beating so hard that I could barely breathe.

As I grew older, I logicized and somehow managed to make myself believe that I was no longer afraid of the dark. However, inside my heart, I always knew that this wasn't completely true. I was distracting my mind every time my phobia started coming on the surface but that didn't imply it was gone for good.

After receiving initiation into Reiki, my phobia came back in full force. I couldn't get even a minute of sleep for almost a week. It would only be after daybreak that I would manage to get a little rest. To add to my woes another health condition I had for a while, allergic rhinitis, came to the surface with full force.

Every time I developed allergic rhinitis, I would be so sick that it would be impossible for me to get out of bed for 5-7 days. That one time it was worse than ever. I called my teacher up and shared what all I was going through. She assured me that there was nothing to worry about and soon I would be fine.

I decided to trust her and continued my practice. It wasn't easy as I was questioning everything. I wasn't even sure if there really is anything known as 'life force energy.' Even if it is there, how was it going to heal me? What I did know was that every time I gave myself Reiki, I felt deeply relaxed and my extremely active mind also managed to remain calm for a certain period of time.

Believe it or not, at the end of the 21-day period, I was a completely different person altogether. No, not all my problems completely disappeared but I was happy and calm. This was a great achievement for someone who had suffered from severe depression for almost 10 years.

I kept practicing and my life kept changing for good. I know that the idea of everything getting amplified initially might be difficult one to accept but trust me, if you decide to take this incredible journey into the world of healing, you will be amazed by how much you and your life has changed. We don't get rid of our fears by denying they exist. We get rid of them by facing them. Through Reiki you can not only face all your health issues and life problems, you can release them to reveal a blank slate on which you can write a new life script.

EXPERIENCING REIKI

If you are not ready to become a Reiki practitioner, you can still receive Reiki healing and study it from afar. In this way, Reiki is like a massage: we all can rub our own muscles when we experience discomfort, but we only get to the core of our discomfort in the hands of a professional.

Receiving Reiki is incredibly relaxing. For the entire duration of the session, you are fully clothed and are laying comfortably on either an elevated massage table or on a blanket on the floor (with head and lower back cushions as needed). Many practitioners encourage their clients to place a blanket over them, since Reiki can often feel like a cold or warm and cozy burst of energy that immediately leaves one feeling at peace (and sleepy).

Once you are settled in and laying down, the practitioner will then ask you a series of questions about what brought you to receive Reiki and if you have any medical or emotional needs for this particular session to focus on. Some Reiki practitioners are also psychics, mediums or intuitives and may also ask you for permission to receive information that may be helpful to your healing experience (such as ask your angels or guides for support in your healing, receive messages or visions about your future, or whatever their specialty may be). Additionally, the Reiki healer may ask you if or how you would like to use supplemental forms of healing during the session, such as essential oils, incense, music, sound healing, or guided meditation. Lastly, the Reiki healer will ask if you prefer that they conduct the healing hand positions lightly touching or hovering over your body. Once you are ready to begin the Reiki healing session, the healer will sit or stand at the top of your head and ask that you gently close your eyes and relax.

Whether we are aware of it or not, consistently or inconsistently, we are all radio towers that are picking up on energy and energetic transmissions in and around us at all times. Since Reiki is universal energy, and we are the signal tower, during the healing session, we may or may not "feel" Reiki in a specific area or throughout our body. This is an important disclaimer to address because there is often a misconception about how a Reiki session "should" "feel". Even if we may not feel a particular expected sensation, it does not mean that Reiki didn't come through or that we are not healed.

Additionally, we may experiencing healing in unexpected ways and in areas of our body that we didn't anticipate that may be related to the particular ailment or discomfort we initially want to address. Remember: the miracle of Reiki is that it intuitive goes where it is needed, devoid of any necessary explanation.

If you do feel sensations, they may also be different for each Reiki session you receive and may also differ from healer to healer as well. You may feel heat, warmth, tingling, coolness, frigid cold, pins and needles or feeling like there are multiple hands "combing" through your energy field. You may also have other types of sensations and experiences, such as sleepiness (even falling completely asleep for the session, which is very common), yawning, burping, hiccupping, stomach growling/gurgling, thirst, bleary eyes, a refreshed and renewed sense of calm, giggling, and peace of mind. Additionally, some individuals experience vivid imagery, messages, colors nad reams

If you are a Reiki practitioner healing another person, you will also feel sensations in your hands as you conduct the energy session. This phenomenon is called "Reiki Hands". Reiki Hands means that your hands are superconductors of reiki energy and therefore are enabling the passage of massive amounts of energy through them and into your client's physical and spiritual body. As a result, your hands may also feel oscilating temperatures of extreme heat, warmth, coolness, tingling, tickling – and – basically any sensation that your client may also be experiencing.

Even if you do not feeling anything as Reiki practitioner, you must trust that the Reiki is still "on" and flowing through, no matter what. Remember that prior to your experience, knowledge and practice of Reiki, it always surrounded and was with you so there is no need to be hard on yourself for not feeling or seeing it the way you want to for your self or with a client.

Chapter 2 - The Five Principles of Reiki

Healing is powerful only when we embrace purity in our words, actions and conduct. The purer we become, rising above the five vices, the more potent our healing experiences will be.

Dr. Usui developed the five Reiki principles in order help each Reiki practitioner transform from the inside out. When we change from the inside, our experiences in the outside world change as well. Outer reality is only an extended manifestation of inner reality.

The best thing about the five Reiki principles is that these are daily pledges that you must take every morning when you start your day. The mind loves timelines and clearly cut-out goals. It is easier to give up on anger for one day than it is to get our minds to accept the idea of giving up on anger for the rest of our lives. Yet one tiny step taken every day can add to an entire life of transformation.

Every morning, right after waking up, you must say these five principles out aloud to yourself. You can even stick these on your bedroom wall or on your desk. Having them in front of your eyes all the time will help you remain connected to the idea of following these principles. Every time, you find yourself falling in the trap of negativity, you can read these principles and remind yourself what your goal is (to heal your body, mind and spirit).

Here are the full ideals and principles of Reiki, as created, taught and practiced by Dr. Usui:

The secret art of inviting happiness

The miraculous medicine of all diseases

> Just for today, do not anger
>
> Do not worry and be filled with gratitude
>
> Devote yourself to your work. Be kind to people.
>
> Every morning and evening, join your hands in prayer.
>
> Pray these words to your heart
>
> And chant these words with your mouth.

However, following these principles religiously will not only heal you from the inside out but they would also transform your relationships with others. So let's quickly capitulate the 5 Reiki principles here:

PRINCIPLE 1 - JUST FOR TODAY, I WILL NOT BE ANGRY

No other emotion is as toxic and paralyzing as anger. Anger might give you a false sense of power but, in truth, it is your greatest enemy. Emotion creates a powerful fight or flight response in your body inducing the release of toxic stress hormones in the body. Stress is the root cause of every disease. Also, at an energetic level, anger creates major blockages in the body preventing the free-flow of life force energy. Think about how you feel when you are angry. After the emotional surge has mellowed down, don't you feel completely drained? Besides, anger ruins relationships. It prevents mutual understanding from happening.

While Reiki is a powerful tool to remove anger blockages from the physical and subtle bodies, it cannot work on current anger if it is still occurring. Letting go of anger not only releases one from the shackles of a destructive emotion but it also empowers and enables you to find constructive solutions to difficult problems.

Now, the question is how not to be angry. Well, I would suggest that every time you are angry, instead of focusing on the negative emotions, you can start chanting a mantra. I have personally experienced miracles through this. You can chant the universal mantra 'Om' or if you are initiated into level 2 Reiki practice, then you can chant the Reiki mantra.

Bringing about a shift in focus is key to transforming your anger. So every time you find yourself slipping into the negative pattern of rage and destructive thinking, shift your focus on chanting a mantra. It will not only calm you down but it also has the potential to miraculously transform a negative situation into a positive one.

PRINCIPLE 2 – JUST FOR TODAY, I WILL NOT WORRY

All the world's great religions talk about the root cause of suffering as being man's inability to live in the present. Worry is always in the future and for things that are likely never going to happen. Also, the law of attraction states that what we think, we attract. Do you really want to attract in your life the very things you are worried about? From this moment onwards, remember that you are not 'worrying,' you are actually creating. Your thoughts are your power – you can use them to create a beautiful life or you can use them to create one disaster after another. Trust that only good things will happen and your faith will start manifesting into reality. I know this is not easy so here's a suggestion. Every time you find yourself worrying, write down all your emotions on paper. Allow yourself to feel all your fears and anxiety as you go about writing your letter. Once you have poured your heart out, light a matchstick and burn the letter. Flush it down the toilet with the intention that you are asking the Universe to take it away from you. Do this every single time you feel overwhelmed by your negative emotions.

Also, create a journal and start writing your goals and vision for life. Write it in the present tense as if everything was happening right now. Soon you will experience a dramatic shift in your life as your subconscious will start attracting wonderful things in your life.

PRINCIPLE 3 – JUST FOR TODAY I WILL BE GRATEFUL

Gratitude is a powerful emotion. It is the master key to unlocking the door of manifestation. The more gratitude you express for all the wonderful things you have been blessed with, the more those things are going to grow in your life. Apply this principle and you will be proven right without any doubt.

You can start maintaining a gratitude journal wherein you write 10 or more things that you are grateful for every night. Obviously, you can do this any time of the day but incorporating any kind of program for positive programming works best during the first hour or so of waking up and before going to sleep. The doorways of the subconscious are wide open during this period and whatever you are going to put into it would have a deep impact on your experience of life.

Also, one of the most powerful principles of manifestation is to become grateful in advance for what you are trying to manifest. Gratitude is like a powerful magnet which would immediately set the forces of the Universe into bringing into material reality the fulfillment of your heart's deepest desires.

PRINCIPLE 4 – JUST FOR TODAY, I WILL DO MY WORK HONESTLY

Each one of us can only have what is truly our share. We might sometimes feel clever stealing a piece of someone else's pie but remember that we have to pay for everything one way or the other. You can only have what is truly yours. Even if you don't snatch someone else's pie, the pie would eventually come to you if you are destined to receive it.

Live with honesty and work with integrity. Even if you feel you aren't being rewarded for your efforts, trust that you would be eventually. It is the law of the Universe that every good deed will be rewarded. Sometimes it takes time but it is destined to come.

PRINCIPLE 5 – JUST FOR TODAY, I WILL BE KIND TO EVERY LIVING THING

Kindness heals not only the giver but the receiver. Kindness is a balm that can soothe everyone's wounds. Even if not physically, we are all psychically wounded in some way or the other living on this dimension of duality. When we give kindness, it comes back to us manifold. I have a simple principle for this: never do to anyone what you wouldn't like for yourself or as Jesus said it, "Do unto others as you would have them do unto you."

Start by being kind and compassionate to those around you. Treat them the way you would like them to treat you. You will be amazed by how deeply content and happy this one thing would make you. Eventually, your circle of kindness will naturally start extending to all living beings. Every day, just pledge to live with greater compassion towards all living beings. Your life will become filled with love, gentleness and kindness.

Chapter 3 - The Importance of Initiation

The concept of initiation is a common one in Asian spiritual practices. Almost every spiritual practice is given through a teacher-disciple relationship. The teacher initiates his disciple into a practice, ceremoniously marking the 'beginning' or initiation of the disciple into a new way of life.

But the question is do you really need an initiation? If Reiki is all about using the Universal life force energy then can't you yourself tap into this energy and start healing yourself right away?

It is hard to explain the process of initiation at a purely logical level as it is, at the core, a mystical experience. The process of initiation cannot be explained in words. It is an experience and an experience can be understood only after one has had that experience.

After initiation, almost every person I have ever known reports feeling a greater sense of calmness and peace. It is an exchange of energy between the master and the student. Energy cannot be seen but it can certainly be experienced. During the initiation practice, the master transfers a part of his meditative energy to the student. People report experiencing dramatic changes in their life and major shifts in perception after the initiation process.

Therefore, to make a long answer short, initiation is indeed a necessity. Why? I think it is best to discover the answer for yourself. You will certainly understand the 'why' after going through the process.

Chapter 4 – Choosing the Right Practitioner

Whether you are interested in receiving Reiki healing treatments or receiving Reiki attunements so you can become the healer, it is imperative that you choose the right healer and/or Master who aligns with your values, needs, and curiosities on your journey with Reiki. Every Reiki practitioner is different: they will have a different method of working with Reiki, may specialize in specific physical and/or emotional healings, and some may be more traditional than others. The following are a few key considerations to keep in mind on your search for the perfect Reiki practitioner for you:

Engage With Them

Chances are that a significant chunk of your research so far has been online. Although first impressions are often everyone's first go-to when making a decision, keep in mind that it is easy to curate a certain "look" or "appeal" meant to attract certain types of customers online. That said, push yourself to go the extra mile and engage with your potential Reiki practitioner in a deeply interpersonal way. You won't have a good sense of this person's personality, demeanor, and the type of energy that they bring to you in your conversation about Reiki. It's important to gauge how you and your potential Reiki practitioner interact and communicate so that you pick the best fit for you.

Trust Your Intuition

Once you're able to speak with a few potential candidates, it might be hard to come to a single choice. Depending on the type of experience you want, especially if it Is your first time receiving Reiki or are considering an attunement, each practitioner probably offers different pros and cons that are weighing your decision. Since Reiki is an investment of your time, money, and energy, it is tempting to spend a lot of time thinking about making the "right" decision. There is merit in not over-thinking it as well: trust your gut. If it feels right, it feels right. Even if the cost, location, or other factors might make you cringe slightly, your Reiki experience with your practitioner is invaluable. Since Reiki is all about energy, if you feel that the energy is perfect with a particular candidate, go for it.

Traditional vs. Non-Traditional Methods

There are many different types and styles of Reiki methods beyond the traditional Usui system that many practitioners use. If you are first starting out with your Reiki experience, you might want to consider choosing a practitioner who uses the Usui method. If you are a little more curious about Reiki and are generally open minded about the different styles of energy healing, you are free and welcome to have your first Reiki experience with a practitioner who has an alternative style and/or approach to healing.

The Experience

Practitioners have different preferences for how they like to give and, in the case of a Reiki master, teach and attune others to Reiki. Some practitioners prefer a one-on-one private session, whereas others thrive in a group setting. If a particular candidate doesn't disclose their preferred environment, be sure to ask so that you are getting the best Reiki experience possible.

Usually, Reiki healing takes place in a wellness center, rental wellness room, and even in a spare room in the practitioner's home. Each of these environments offers a different kind of experience. Wellness centers and rental wellness rooms are usually located in very quiet neighborhoods and are decorated with light colors, full of plants or crystals, and are well maintained since they are shared spaces for clients and practitioners. In this setting, it will feel very curated, clean, and welcoming. If your practitioner offers services from their own home, you can expect a much more intimate and personal experience since they are also offering you're their personal hospitality in their personal space. Some individuals feel more comfortable depending on either of these settings, so it is important to make sure that your Reiki experience is in your ideal environment.

Values, Spiritual Philosophy, and Approaches to Healing

Another important consideration to take into account for your Reiki experience is your alignment with your healers' values, spiritual philosophy and/or their approach to healing. Take note of the kind of language and beliefs they have in their approach and make sure that they align with your own so that you do not feel any doubt, skepticism, uncertainty, or disagreement with your practitioner's beliefs or pedagogical values and approaches to Reiki healing.

Their Credentials and Work History

Most practitioners have a personal website that details client testimonials and a resume that details how long they have been healing and working with others in group and one-on-

one sessions. It would be worth your while to see if your practitioner has reviews on Google or Yelp, for example, so that you can look into any feedback that might not have been included on their website (i.e. more recent feedback, or negative feedback in particular). If their work history includes residencies and group sessions at healing or wellness centers, you can call these locations and ask their managers or owners what their impression and experience has been with your practitioner.

Chapter 5 – How to Receive Reiki Attunements

The Importance and Necessity of Receiving Reiki Attunements

Although universal life energy, or Reiki, is always all around us, everywhere and in everything, it requires a special initiation process for those who wish to readily access and harness it for healing and manifestation work. This initiation process, known as reijuu, is a special ceremony conducted by a Reiki Master. In this ceremony, the initiate receives several attunements (which are secret energy seals that the Reiki Master seals into your hands and energy field) . These attunements are sealed in the initiate for life and allow them to easily access and work with Reiki for their self or other healing practices.

Who Can Receive Attunements

Anyone can receive Reiki attunements. There are no special perquisites, requirements to receive attunements. One doesn't need a comprehensive understanding of Reiki, it's history, it's uses; and, in fact, you could arguably just walk on in from the street and get an attunement without any in-depth knowledge of Reiki. You can be in any form of physical and mental health to receive a Reiki attunement. There are no age limits for Reiki attunements: all are welcome to understand how energy works (and, many believe that the younger that this concept is understood and mastered, the better!). All you need is a general understanding and acceptance that all things, time and matter are energy that we all have the ability to work with, redirect, and reshape these energetic forces for the highest good of all involved.

Reiki is not a religion or a spiritual practice, it is simply a healing modality. The ceremony has no religious elements or traditions. It is simply the process by which you receive the ability to access Reiki through a series of secret symbols that a Reiki Master places in your energetic field and in the palms of your hands. As you will learn further in this chapter, only a Reiki Master can provide attunements.

Preparing for Attunement

The reiki attunement process is intense, impactful and transformative for the recipient on the energetic, emotional, and physical layers of their well being. It is strongly advised that the recipient wears comfortable, light colored clothing for the day of their attunement process and drinks plenty of water. Since a tremendous amount of energy is transmuted upon the recipient (and, in some cases, the recipient may begin practicing their newly acquired Reiki techniques as soon as they are attuned), keeping hydrated is especially important to prevent exhaustion and fatigue.

Since Reiki can stir up unresolved emotions, it is also important to make time to process the Reiki attunement just before and after. Many Reiki Masters strongly advise that the first few days after the attunement process are the most intense, and therefore, require a significant amount of intentional rest periods. Reiki initiates need to make sure they drink a sufficient amount of water, rest for subsequent periods of time, and give themselves space and permission to process any memories, emotions, feelings and/or physical sensations that come up throughout the attunement process.

The Attunement

The attunement process is considered very sacred and it is therefore secret. If you've been interested in receiving Reiki attunements, you'll find that there is virtually no information on the *how* of the attunement ceremony. Instead, you'll learn about the instructor, whether it is a 1-1 or group attunement process, and what to wear, bring, etcetera. You would also learn that not only do you receive the attunements, but also learn how to give Reiki through level-specific hand positions, symbols, and other techniques for healing yourself and others. Since Reiki can operate across the energetic and physical plane, attunements can take place either in-person or via remote conferencing from a Reiki Master.

> In-Person Attunements
> In-person attunements can take the format of either a one-on-one session or as a group. In either scenario, the Reiki Master will give you the attunements for your Level and will show you the specific healing strategies, symbols and hand positions for that Level. One-on-one sessions typically range from 3-4 hours long over the course of one to two days, whereas group sessions usually take 5-6 hours long.

> Remote Attunements
> Since Reiki can flow through time and space, attunements do not have to be geographic-specific or even take place in person. Reiki Masters are able to attune their students through phone calls, skype, googlehangout, and even facetime sessions. Attunements require an interpersonal exchange, so be leery of any videos, tweets, and even images that claim to attune you simply by clicking on that particular media. Authentic remote attunements require live, interpersonal interactions in order to work.

Level I, Level II and Reiki Master Ceremonies

Depending on your personal experience with Reiki, there are three different attunement and practitioner levels: Level I, II, and III. In Level I, you are attuned to receive four different symbols so that you can use Reiki. In Level II, you are not only attuned to receive three additional symbols but you are able to use these three symbols in your own practice. The Level III attunement process is known as the "Reiki Master" level: this is the level that not only attunes you to two additional symbols, but also teaches you all of the symbols necessary to attune others through Reiki. Simply going through the Level I and II attunement phases do not qualify you with the ability to attune another person. In fact, the instructional content and ability to provide others with Reiki attunements is only possible through completing Level I, II and III of Reiki

Healing Crisis

Receiving Reiki attunements is a heavy, energetic activity for the physical body. As a result, your body may tailspin into an emotional and physical detoxing process for at least 30 days after receiving Reiki attunements. This is known as the "healing crisis". Since Reiki energy helps the body achieve homeostasis, receiving the Reiki attunements will also invoke this same response in the initiate. Typical symptoms of a healing crisis include: coming down with a cold, sinus pressure, fever, lack of appetite, lethargy, or light headedness This is a completely natural part of the Reiki process and it lets the initiate know that Reiki is flowing through their body to heal them so they can be a stronger practitioner for themselves and others.

The healing crisis can also align itself (and typically does) with the 21 Day Pledge. Since the mind and body are undergoing a radical transformation during this time, it is no surprise that our physical and emotional wellbeing physically shifts also and presents itself as illness. During this time, we are also exposed to habits, thought patterns, and beliefs that may have been hindering our growth and from reaching our fullest potential. Take care to observe this time in your transition to becoming a Reiki practitioner, as there are messages in this deeply personal healing for you to learn from and work on through Reiki.

Chapter 6 - The 7 Chakras

There are 7 chakras in the human body. While they are not visible to the physical eyes, any person with clairvoyant or intuitive abilities can see them. Each chakra appears as a revolving vortex, like a wheel, of energy. When one has a too many unresolved emotions or issues in life, these chakras become blocked. A clairvoyant person will be able to perceive this as a cloud of dense black energy in the affected area.

Diseases first occur in the subtle bodies as the chakras become blocked. Think about it; a lot of people complain about feeling an ache in the heart but when they get an ECG, nothing comes out in it. However, this person continues to feel the ache and finally, one day, after a few months, the diseased heart condition shows up in test reports. Isn't this true?

The good news is that regular practice of Reiki removes all blockages enabling a free flow of life force energy. Reiki flows in and out of the physical and spiritual body, leaving us feeling lighter and balanced in both areas of our lives so that we prevent and heal all the root causes of disease and illness. Since the root cause of every disease is psychosomatic, if you stay true to your practice, you will certainly be in the best of health for life.

CHAKRA 1 – THE BASE/ROOT CHAKRA

Located at the base of spine, this is the first chakra. Symbolized by a deep red color and a lotus with four petals, it forms the foundation of the entire chakra system. This chakra is associated with survival or with the basic necessities of life: food, security and shelter. Traumatic experiences wherein we experienced any kind of threat to our survival needs could lead to major blockages in the root chakra. This blockage can manifest in the form of irrational fear of loss, a deep feeling of insecurity, spinal health issues, etc.

The root chakra is associated with the earth element. Since earth is heavy and solid, when in balance, this chakra gives us a sense of stability and security.

Chakra 2 – The Sacral chakra

The second chakra is located in the lower abdomen region between the genitals and the navel. Symbolized by the color orange and a lotus with six petals, this chakra is associated with the water element. Therefore, it is associated with liquid-related bodily functions: circulation, urinary function, reproduction and sexuality. The sacral chakra is the seat of our sexuality. It governs our sensory experiences, emotions, creativity, pleasure, nurturance and movement. Sexual abuse and traumatic sexual experiences could cause serious blockages in the sacral chakra. The individual might also be overly sensitive to other people and their emotions which could result in frequent dramatic emotional episodes. When the second chakra is open and functioning properly, the individual experiences a heightened sense of creativity and sensual/creative awareness.

Chakra 3 - Solar Plexus

The solar plexus is located at the bottom of the rib cage in the abdominal region. Symbolized by a yellow colored lotus with ten petals, this chakra governs our actions, our sense of personal power and our vitality. It represents the fire element and governs our will and desire to take actions. At the physical level, it is associated with the function of digestion. Any blockages in this chakra can manifest in the form of stomach ailments, digestive troubles, ulcers, addiction, diabetes, etc. People with blockages in the solar plexus also tend to suffer from a general lack of energy. The individual might also feel jaded, tired and withdrawn. They could come out as being too serious with little light-heartedness or laughter.

Chakra 4 – The Heart Chakra

Symbolized by a green colored lotus with twelve petals, the heart chakra is associated with the feeling of compassion and love. It is located around the same region where the physical heart exists. Associated with the air element, this chakra is said to be the seat of the Holy Spirit. Traumatic emotional experiences, relationship breakups, betrayal, etc. cause blockages of the heart chakra. When the heart chakra is closed, one might experience a general sense of apathy and a lack of compassion towards others. When the heart chakra is healthy and harmonious, it radiates unconditional love. However, the path of love always begins with self-love and total self-acceptance. With regular practice of Reiki, the practitioner gradually begins to shed all kinds of social conditioning that teach one to practice self-annihilation and self-abnegation.

Chakra 5 – The Throat Chakra

The fifth chakra is symbolized by a bright blue lotus with 16 petals. This chakra, located at the base of the throat, is the seat of communication and creative expression. Associated with the ether element, it is this chakra that facilitates our ability to communicate. One must remember that communication effective communication is a two-way street. It isn't just about our ability to speak but it also relates to our ability to listen. Any kind of blockages in this chakra can result in an inability to express one's thoughts and feelings. On the other extreme end, it could also make a person so verbose that they might find it hard to listen to others. Regular practice of Reiki awakens us to our highest creative potential as it removes energetic blockages from the throat chakra.

CHAKRA 6 – THE THIRD EYE

Located in-between the eyebrows, the third eye, is symbolized by an indigo-colored lotus with two petals. When the third eye is awakened, an individual is able to perceive that which lies beyond the five senses. It is the seat of psychic power and awakening the third chakra endows the individual with clairvoyant facilities. The third eye corresponds to the pineal gland and directly affects its functioning. Blockages of the third chakra can manifest as an irrational fear of ghosts or as excess worry of the future. It can also hinder our ability to perceive the truth and process information in any given situation. Regular practice of Reiki can awaken the third chakra enhancing one's intuitive faculties.

CHAKRA 7 – THE CROWN CHAKRA

The crown chakra is located at the top of the head. It is symbolized by a violet-colored lotus with a thousand petals. The crown chakra is the seat of Higher Consciousness. It represents our connection with the Universe. When the crown chakra is fully awakened, the individual experiences enlightenment. In a regular person, there's likely to be some amount of blockages in the crown chakra. It is from this chakra that we draw into our physical and subtle bodies, the life force energy of the Universe. Severe blockages of the crown chakra can result in chronic depression, a feeling of disconnection, lack of direction in life, loneliness, etc. Reiki energy can harmonize all our chakras transforming us into perfect vessels for drawing in the infinite life force energy of the Universe.

Chapter 7 - Reiki Level 1

Every Reiki practitioner begins his practice with self-healing or level 1. The hands-on practice of level 1 is deeply relaxing and grounding. After each Reiki session that you give yourself, you will come out feeling more refreshed and rejuvenated than ever. You must do this practice every day without fail for at least 21-days post initiation. It is going to change your life and you would know how far you have come at the end of the 21-day period.

IMPORTANT THINGS TO REMEMBER:

- Remove all jewelry and watches before starting a Reiki session as metal can interfere with the transmission of energy.
- If you are suffering from any kind of disease, then you must keep taking your regular medications. Reiki will not only enhance the results but will also enable a speedy recovery.
- Fix a time for your practice and stick to it no matter what. You can do it before going to sleep for excellent deep sleep.
- The 21-day period is a period of detox. This detox is likely to take place not only at the physical level but also at an emotional, mental and energetic level. Unwanted emotions and unwanted memories might also come to the surface. You must make a promise to yourself to not quit your practice before the end of 21 days. Trust me, in the end it will be all worthwhile!
- Drink plenty of water throughout the day and maintain a clean diet throughout this period to get maximum benefits.

- Avoid going to parties and crowded places as they can drain your energy while you are going through a critical period of energetic detoxification. Likewise, avoid the company of negative people altogether.

- Keep your intentions pure and your mind focused on what you want. Wish everyone well and good things will come to you as well.

- Reiki is an energy, therefore, it works even on top of clothing.

- You can practice Reiki anywhere and anytime. Whenever, you feel a need, feel free to invoke the Reiki energy and start giving yourself healing.

- Touch yourself with tenderness and love. Look at and feel every part of your body with gentleness and gratitude.

- Inculcate self-love. Treat yourself the way you would like others to treat you.

- Trust that everything is happening for the best and eventually, all the bits and pieces would fit together in perfect harmony.

THE LEVEL 1 PRACTICE

Each session of Reiki must begin with an invocation along with a recitation of the five principles. The invocation will immediately increase your vibrational frequency aligning you with the purest of the pure healing energy of the Universe.

Your teacher will give you the exact words to be used during the invocation. However, it could be something like this:

"Right at this moment, I am invoking the purest light of the Universe in my heart

I have become a perfect channel for the divine love of the Universe

My being, my heart, every part of me, is illuminated by the light of God

As His power flows through me and into me."

After the invocation, gently lie down or sit in a comfortable chair and start placing your hands on the different energy centers.

TREATING OTHERS WITH REIKI LEVEL 1

Right after receiving your initiation, you can immediately start treating others as well. The hand positions are pretty much the same except that they are placed differently on the patient's body.

You can ask your patient to lie down and take deep breaths in order to slip into a relaxed state which would automatically make him more receptive to the healing energy of Reiki.

However, before starting the treatment, you must practice *Kenyoku or dry bathing*. Your teacher will initiate you in the actual practice. It is the practice of disconnecting yourself from all unwanted energies in your surroundings including those that your patient might be harboring. Kenyoku will also help you in transforming all your negative and worrisome thoughts.

Chapter 8 - Reiki Level 2

Level 1 Reiki is geared towards self-healing. In order to become ready for the next level of Reiki, one must have practiced level 1 for the prescribed 21-day period and regularly thereafter. Regular practice of level 1 leads to intense purification which in turn increases one's capacity to receive and channelize the higher vibrations of level 2 Reiki.

Also, the healing and life transformation that takes place after the level 1 practice strengthens one's faith in the healing power of Reiki. Usually, there is a powerful inner knowing when one is truly ready to move forward with the next level of Reiki.

DISTANCE HEALING

Reiki level 2 involves distance healing which means sending healing energy without being bound by the limitations of time and space. Science is beginning to understand this phenomenon. In one research, scientists discovered that electrons separated by a distance of 1.3 km were still able to affect each other. Religion and spirituality has long advocated the fact that we are all One and science is starting to acknowledge the fact that indeed we live in an interconnected universe.

Level 2 Reiki compels us to move beyond our limited understanding of our own Truth. It compels us to embrace that which is eternal and infinite. Even if one starts off with initial skepticism, healing will still take place and when one's faith becomes stronger, healing will be more profound than ever.

After level 2 initiation, the practitioner will once again have to go through a detoxification of 21 days. It is likely that many more buried emotions and suppressed traumatic memories will come up. One must not fear this as everything is coming up to finally get resolved and released.

Post level 2 initiation, the practitioner can heal others from a distance while also having the ability to heal his own circumstances and life problems. No matter how difficult or complicated the situation might seem, Reiki has the power to transform anything and everything.

For self-healing, it is still advisable for the individual to continue practicing the hands-on healing method. The only difference that will happen now is that the results will come about faster and more pronounced than ever.

Again, one must not embark on this journey without receiving initiation from a teacher who is also a sincere practitioner of this Divine healing art.

Chapter 9 - The Three Pillars of Reiki

The five principles of Reiki are closely tied to the three pillars of Reiki. Just like the five pillars, the three pillars of Reiki also appeared to Dr. Usui during his retreat where he discovered the Reiki symbols. The three pillars of Reiki are:

- Gassho
- Reiji-Ho
- Chiryo

Now let us explore these in detail:

Gassho

This is a ritual gesture performed by joining both palms and fingers together in a prayer position. It is frequently used to express respect and gratitude. Gassho helps in focusing the mind by bringing it into the present. This gesture also brings about an instant sense of balance and inner peace. Symbolically, it represents Universal consciousness – the congruence and totality within all of existence.

Gassho Meditation

Dr. Usui recommended the practice of Gassho meditation for 5-20 minutes both morning and evening. He insisted that his students start each Reiki session by first grounding and centering themselves through the practice of Gassho. Here's how to perform the meditation:

- Sit down in a comfortable position keeping your back straight.
- Bring your hands together in the Gassho gesture in front of your chest.

- Close your eyes and breathe deeply.
- Focus your attention at the point where the two middle fingers meet.
- Allow yourself to simply be. If thoughts come, then acknowledge them first and then let them go. Don't resist as what you resist will always persist.
- After 5-20 minutes, rub your palms together and place them on your eyes. Slowly open your eyes making your sure that you don't lose the grounded feeling you have just developed through the practice.

Reiji-Ho

Reiji-Ho refers to a series of rituals performed before starting each Reiki session. Here's how to perform Reiji-Ho:

- Close your eyes and brings your hands together in the Gassho position in front of your chest.
- In your heart, declare the intention to connect with the healing energy of Reiki. Do this three times. If you are initiated into level 2, then use the Reiki symbols.
- Feel the Reiki energy entering through your crown chakra, flowing into your heart center and into your palms.
- Pray for the good health and healing of your patient while stating the intention of serving as a pure vessel for Reiki's healing energy.
- Retaining your hands in the Gassho position, take them to your third eye. Ask Reiki energy to guide your hands to those places where healing is needed.

- Follow your intuition as you give healing to your patient. Your hands will automatically be guided to the right area. You will also know when to move on to the next region. Don't worry about how this is going to happen. Surrender fully to the experience and retain purity of intention.

- Once the healing session has been completed, you will automatically be guided to place your hands on your thighs with the palms facing downward.

- Complete the session by once again bringing your hands together in Gassho.

- Remain detached and don't allow your logic mind to interfere. Trust that the guidance you are receiving is real.

- Also, practice detachment from the outcome. Have faith in the fact that healing is taking place even if the results aren't exactly what you would have wanted.

Chiryo

Chiryo can be literally translated into English as "treatment." For this, the Reiki practitioner places his dominant hand on top of the patient's head praying for the patient's healing while waiting for inspiration to arise. It is important for the practitioner to surrender all thoughts and doubts. Once inspiration comes, the hand will automatically be guided to the right places where healing is needed.

Chapter 10 – Introduction to Alternative Reiki Healing Systems

Although this guide is based on and utilizes the original, traditional Usui Reiki method, there are actually 1,200 different types of Reiki healing styles, based on a total of 10 different branches of Reiki healing treatments. Each of these different Reiki healing systems builds upon the traditional Usui methods and symbols to target a particular type of healing purpose, effect, or alternative energetic approach.

Despite the popularity of Reiki and all of its diverse styles, there is no comprehensive record in existence that lists all 1,200 styles. Listed below are the most popular and well-known alternative Reiki styles and approaches that are well documented, recorded and regularly practiced throughout the Reiki community, listed in order of popularity.

Different Reiki Styles:

Karuna

Derived from the Sanskirt word for compassion, this type of Reiki was developed by Usui Reiki Master and Founder of the International Center for Reiki Training, William Lee Rand in 1995. Karuna is very similar to the traditional Usui Reiki system; in fact, the only difference is that it simply has eight additional symbols developed by Rand based on observations he made during his Reiki Master practice. These symbols allow the practitioner and the recipient of the Reiki to specifically feel more compassion in their spirit, lives and physical bodies, just as the name Karuna suggests.

Rainbow

This style of Reiki descents from one of the original Usui Reiki Masters, Madame Takata, who went on to attune future practitioners in her home state of Hawaii. Rainbow Reiki was developed by Walter Lubek, who is one of Takata's disciples and students.

Kundalini

This method of Reiki is accessed only through Kundalini Yoga practice. Since Kundalini requires the practitioner to access their internal energy systems through the seven chakras, this form of Reiki is only accessed by performing and practicing Kundalini yoga. It is only meant for use during the Kundalini Yoga practice and is meant for the practitioner only.

Osho Neo

Osho Neo was created by Usui Reiki Master Rajneesh, who was also an avid Kundalini Reiki practitioner. Rajneesh wanted to create a new style of reiki that combined the traditional Usui symbols with the principals of the chakra healing system and techniques in Kundalini Yoga.

Blue Star Celestial

This form of Reiki healing is rooted in ancient Egyptian energetic healing techniques, which are all based on the principal star constellations that the pyramids are built under. The practitioner must have an astute understanding of the cosmologically based energetic healing systems of the Egyptians in order to practice this form of Reiki.

Chios Energy Healing

This healing system combines the Kundalini chakra healing traditions and systems with aura healing techniques. Unlike traditional Kundalini Reiki, Chios energy healing can be performed without doing yoga. Since the aura is also healed in this process, Chios Energy Healing is incredibly thorough.

Celtic

This style of Reiki combines ancient Celtic symbols and energetic healing techniques with the Usui Reiki symbols and strategies. The effect is incredibly grounding and soothing. Celtic Reiki is often practiced in woodsy and/or forest environments.

Karmic

This form of Reiki incorporates elements of distance healing in Usui Level II Reiki with the Hindu principals of karma. Karmic reiki specifically explores and heals one's various past lives and present actions in order to ensure that significant lessons are learned, healed, and new, growth-driven and positive experiences are established in order to help repair one's evolving karma in this life time and in the next.

Raku Kei

Raku Kei is believed to actually be a sect of traditional Usui Reiki. Raku Kei includes several new symbols and self-healing techniques that were not passed down from Usui himself. Raku Kei is a series of technique found in Usui's various personal archives and it is considered to be a critical supplement to the traditional Usui Reiki system. Many traditional Usui Reiki Masters have advocated that Raku Kei is officially recognized and incorporated into the traditional Usui Reiki attunement and instructional process as a result.

Sacred or Violet Flame

The Sacred Flame (also known as the Violet Flame) is very similar to the traditional Usui Reiki method; however, this form of Reiki require seven additional attunements for the practitioner and it also gives full license to the Master to create their own symbols. It is believed that the large number of Reiki styles is attributed to this method in the Sacred/Violet Flame Reiki practice as a result.

How to Practice Non-Usui Reiki Systems

Almost all of these Reiki systems require special attunements and/or guidance from their respective Reiki Masters. The easiest and fastest way to get information on how you can learn and practice these different systems Is to conduct a comprehensive search on Google.com or join Reiki practitioner Facebook groups and ask to speak with a Reiki Master from one of these divisions to attune and teach you their methods for healing.

Chapter 11 - Level I Self-Healing Techniques

Reiki practitioners from all types of beginning and advanced backgrounds will all advocate for the importance of regular, self-healing with Reiki. Maintaining a regular, daily self-healing practice reaps many benefits for the practitioner, including: a stronger immune system, feeling more peaceful and less prone to stress, feeling balanced and calm, and, a stronger intuition and relationship with Reiki, the body, and the variety of hand positions for effective Reiki experiences. Self-healing not only allows the practitioner to maintain a regular healing practice for themselves, but the continuous dedication to this work allows them to self-experiment with new techniques and methods that they can then transfer to a client. Ultimately, maintaining a strong, regular self- healing practice is beneficial for both the practitioner and their future clients in the long run.

Preparing Yourself for Self-Healing

Self-healing can happen anywhere and at any time, so long as you are able to comfortably focus on what you're doing. Some practitioners like to do self-healing in public settings such as their commute or in a park, whereas others prefer to recreate similar environments for their clients: in a quiet, private, and meditative space dedicated specifically for Reiki healing. Self-healing simply requires time and concentration, so choose an environment that allows you to fully embrace both of these qualities so you can be fully present with your self-healing practice.

Duration and Frequency

Self-healing traditionally takes 30 minutes; however, with practice, you may find that you will take the amount of time that works best for you. You can practice self-healing as many times as you'd like throughout the day: the only minimum is that you practice at least once a day!

Positive Effectives of Regular Self Healing Practice

Just like exercising regularly, self-healing on a daily basis has several emotional and physical benefits. Regular Reiki healing can support with healing pre-existing conditions such as stress, anxiety, depression, nervousness, bloating, acute pain, cuts, bruises, and muscle tensions and sprains. Regular Reiki self-healing keeps the body's cells, tissues, and organs feeling cleansed, balanced, and repaired.

Self-Healing Hand Positions and Techniques

Self-healing techniques are based on the traditional Usui method hand positions. Over time, many Reiki practitioners have created slight modifications based on what works for them over time. As you learn the self-healing techniques below, know that with time and practice, you are also likely to create your own set of techniques that work best for you.

In each of these positions, your palms will be touching your body. Please note that you are to place your palms in a straight line so that your fingertips are touch each other (do not place your palms on top of each other).

First Position – Palms Over Each Eye

In this position, you place the palms of your hands over each eye. This position allows for healing of the eyes, sinuses, brain, pituitary gland, pineal gland and the third eye chakra. This is the position used for eye strain, eye stress, headaches, migraines, anxiety, stress, fevers, allergies, colds and flus.

Second Position – Palms on Each Side of the Neck

In this position, you place each of your palms on either side of your neck, just slightly underneath the ears. This position allows you to bring healing to your lungs, esophagus, pulmonary arteries, lymph nodes, vocal chords, thyroid, and the throat chakra. This is the position associated with healing lymphatic and thyroid disorders, artery and heart issues, asthma, laryngitis, fear of public speaking, and ensuring that your communications are clear and well heard.

Third Position – Palms Over the Sternum / Breastbone (Just Below Collarbone)

This position focuses on bringing healing to the upper lungs, heart, thymus gland (which is the gland responsible for stress), breasts, and the heart chakra. This is the position used to healing and treating asthma, breathing issues, pneumonia, heart issues and disease, breast cancer, chronic stress and/or anxiety, and matters related to relationships, self-love, love, and passion.

Fourth Position – Palms Over the Chest (Between Collarbone and Bellybutton)

In this position, you place your palms directly over your heart and chest area. This position brings continued healing to the same areas described in the third position.

Fifth Position – Palms Over the Belly Button

In this position, you place both of your palms directly over the bellybutton. This position brings healing to the stomach, pancreas, kidneys, gallbladder, liver, and is associated with the solar plexus chakra. This is the position to use when you are treating any health issues related to the digestive tract, liver, and kidneys. Additionally, since the solar plexus chakra is associated with creativity, this is a good position to work with if you are experiencing any blockages or lack of inspiration.

Sixth Position – Palms Under the Belly Button, Above the Groin

In this position, you need to place the palms of your hand just above your groin, but slightly below the bellybutton. This allows you to bring Reiki healing to the small intestines, large intestines, and colon. These positions not only bring additional healing for the digestive track, but also support with healing needs for anyone afflicted with celiac or irritable bowel syndrome.

Seventh Position – Palms On the Groin Area

In this final position, you are to place the palms of your hands on either side of your groin. This position brings additional healing to the digestive and urinary systems and also heals any issues related to the reproductive organs, hormones, and pregnancy. This area of the body is also associated with the root chakra, so this healing position is also helpful for healing matters associated with security, safety, and financial opportunities.

Guided Meditation for Self-Healing: 30-45 Minutes Long

You might want to read this aloud and record yourself so you can play back this meditation and follow along! Enjoy:

Close your eyes and slowly breathe in and out, softening your neck, your shoulders, breathing deeply and allowing your arms, hands, lower back, ankles and feet relax. Take slow, deep breathes as you gently feel yourself relaxing and easing into a calm and peaceful state.

Inhale deeply and tightly clasp your palms together just above your heart. Breathe in, slowly calling Reiki into your palms using the methods that feel most comfortable to you. Focus your intent on providing yourself with a loving, healing, and warm Reiki session for your highest good. Ask Reiki to free your spiritual and physical bodies of any negative energies that are holding you back. Breathe deeply, and allow Reiki to flow and pulse in the palms of your hands. You are ready to begin to heal yourself.

First, you will scan your aura. Feel your hands slowly guide themselves around your energetic field, hovering them around your body, beginning with the top of your head and guiding them all the way down to your toes. Feel how your hands burn and cool as you gently hover them over your body, being mindful of detecting any blockages or chords in your energetic field. Observe what you feel in your aura, and how your hands feel when you detect any challenging energies in your aura. Do you feel your hands are more inclined to stay in a certain area for a longer amount of time for some reason?

Take a deep breath in, and with your palms, pretend you are smoothing your aura, like it is a big blanket whose wrinkles you want to smooth over. Keep the flow of Reiki strong in your palms as you smooth your hands back and forth throughout your energy field. Now, draw your hands back to the areas of any blockages you identified earlier. Breathe deeply and keep your hands over any of these areas, observing the color, emotions, names, people, places, sounds, shapes, and textures of these blockages. Hovering your hands around your energetic field, wash your body completely once more with Reiki energy.

When you are done, bring your hands to the top of your head, breathing deeply and guiding energy to swoop up around and back down your body, all the way to your toes. You are now ready to begin to send Reiki throughout the body. Inhale deeply, imaging that bright, white healing light is coming into your whole body. As you exhale, breathe out the colors, sounds, feelings, and textures that each of your blockages held. Exhale them deeply from your body, feeling them slowly release through your breath.

Guide your hands from the top of your head, feeling Reiki energy permeate there and through your body. Slowly guide your hands down your head, passing your third eye, cupping your ears gently, placing your hands over eyes and then under your chin and ears. Breathe deeply as you feel Reiki energy flow throughout your head, healing the tissues, glands, energies and emotions there.

Guide your hands down your neck, paying attention to gently delivering energy through the sides and back of your neck, slowly moving down to your shoulders, collarbone, and the top of your chest. Breathe deeply, feeling reiki energy guide itself here and through your heart center.

Guide your hands from your chest to your abdomen, placing your hands above, at, and below your navel, breathing deeply. Feel Reiki energy flow throughout the core of your body, flowing through your center, healing the tissues, muscles, organs, energies and emotions there. Breathe deeply, and when you are ready, continue guiding your hands to your hips, thighs, knees, calves, ankles, balls of your feet, and down and out through your toes.

Breathe deeply as you feel Reiki move through the lower half of your body, which carries you every day. Feel healing light nourish the muscles, blood vessels, joints, and any stiffness, aches, and energies there. Give each of your toes a gentle tug, letting them know you are rooted, that you are held. Guide your hands back to your ankles, them move them up to your elbows, wrists, and fingertips. Feel Reiki energy cleanse the muscles, vessels, tensions and energies there. Give your fingers a gentle tug, thanking them for helping you guide energy today, yesterday, and tomorrow.

When you are done, allow your hands to freely guide themselves where you feel you need Reiki. During a Reiki session, sometimes our hands want to rest themselves on a particular part of the body that needs more attention than others. If you are not sure where to put your hands, you can gently rest them on your abdomen and visualize and feel Reiki flowing through you, like a steady stream of light.

Slowly pass Reiki energy throughout your body as many times as you feel you need, using this same process with the hand positions or keeping your hands resting on your abdomen, exhaling out any remaining blockages. If you feel that you are still stuck, imagine that this energy is a ball, or a rope, or sword that you need to gentle pull out of your body. Try pulling this energy lovingly out of your body, thanking it for it's work, and asking for it to never return.

If you have not encountered any blockages, continue breathing in and out, sending Reiki all throughout your body by placing your hands where you feel drawn to most. When you feel that you are full of light, breathe deeply and take in the feelings that Reiki has given you throughout. Bring your hands back to your heart center, breathing deeply, allowing the healing sensations to continue to flow through your body.

When you are ready to come back to the room, slowly breathe in and out, relishing in the peace that you and reiki have brought. Thank reiki for providing you with a healing experience that served your highest good. Close your connection with Reiki. You are now down with this healing session.

Observe how these techniques have felt for you and, if they align with your existing observations throughout your healing journey. You may even want to refer to any notes you recorded when you first explored your mind/body connection and your earlier self-healing sessions to see if these observations align or are alleviated through self-healing with Reiki over time.

This long self-healing session is an excellent exercise to incorporate into your Reiki routine. Practicing this self-healing exercise frequently has many benefits: First, you will be providing yourself with consistent healing; Second, it will become easier to guide the energy; And third, your healing sessions will start to strengthen and have greater effect.

After a few times following along, see if you can practice without the audio and slow down each of the healing movements to make the session last 30 minutes. Each time you revisit this self-healing session, observe how your hands will gradually begin to guide themselves to where your body most needs Reiki to flow. Reflect on how, if at all, these findings have changed for you as you regularly heal yourself with Reiki. Enjoy.

Guided Meditation for Self-Healing: 5-15 Minutes Long

Close your eyes and gently slow your breathing. Take a few deep breathes in and out, softening your neck, your shoulders, breathing deeply and allowing your arms, hands, lower back, ankles and feet to relax. Take slow, deep breathes as you gently feel yourself relaxing and easing into a calm and peaceful state.

Inhale deeply, rubbing your palms together above your heart. Breathe in, slowly bringing Reiki to your palms, and feel Reiki slowly coming into your hands. Ask that it heal you for your highest good, ask that this light cleanse and balance your emotional, spiritual and your physical body and free it of any impurities, blockages, and darkness from within you. Breathe deeply, being mindful of how Reiki feels in your hands.

When you feel that your flow of Reiki is especially strong, bring your hands to crown of your head, breathing deeply and guiding energy to swoop up around and back down your body, all the way to your toes.

Guide your hands from the top of your head, feeling Reiki energy permeate there and through your body. Breathe deeply as you feel Reiki energy flow throughout your head, healing the tissues, glands, energies and emotions there.

Guide your hands down your neck, paying attention to gently sending energy through the sides and back of your neck, slowly moving down to your shoulders, collarbone, and the top of your chest. Breathe deeply, feeling reiki energy guide itself here and through your heart center.

Guide your hands from your chest to your abdomen, placing your hands above, at, and below your navel, breathing deeply. Feel Reiki energy flow throughout the center of your body, healing the tissues, organs, muscles, energies and emotions there. Breathe deeply, and when you are ready, continue guiding your hands to your hips, knees, calves, ankles, balls of your feet, and out through your toes. Guide your hands back to your ankles, them move them up to your elbows, wrists, and finger tips. Feel Reiki energy cleanse the muscles, vessels, tensions and energies there.

When you are done, allow your hands to guide themselves where you feel you need to to guide Reiki. Slowly pass Reiki energy throughout your body as many times as you feel you need, using this same process, exhaling out any blockages you may feel.

When you are ready to come back to the room, slowly breathe in and out, relishing in the peace that you and reiki have brought. Thank reiki for providing you with a healing experience that served your highest good. You may now close your connection with Reiki.

This quick self-healing session is a good alternative if you are short on time; however, it should not be used as a substitute all the time for a full body healing session. Each of the major body points that were healed in this session are the most basic, key areas. If you are still pressed on time, you can only focus on one area of the body instead of healing your entire self. Enjoy.

Chapter 12: Level I Healing Techniques for Others

Preparing for Healing Another as a Level I Reiki Practitioner

All Reiki Level I practitioners have the ability to heal others and themselves. The hand positions and techniques are based on the traditional Usui methods; however, just like with maintaining a regular self-healing practice, the more you heal on others, you will come to have your own adjusted hand positions and methods that work best for you and your clients.

Preparing Your Client for Reiki

No matter the setting, your client can sit, stand, or lay down. Both of you can agree what is most comfortable for them before you begin. Be sure to ask about any pre-existing or current health and/or emotional conditions so that you can bring extra attention to the parts of the body that may need additional love and healing. Before your client comes in for Reiki, make sure that they are wearing comfortable clothes and drink a sufficient amount of water.

Duration and Frequency

Reiki traditionally takes 30 minutes; however, depending on your client's needs, it may take an hour to an hour and a half at most. The longer the session, the more your client will need to take care of themselves after the session by drinking lots of water, avoiding caffeine and alcohol, and allowing their bodies and minds to peacefully adjust to the balance and peace of mind that Reiki can bring.

Healing Hand Positions and Techniques

These healing hands techniques are based on the traditional Usui method hand positions. Over time, many Reiki practitioners have created slight modifications based on what works for them and their clients over time. As you learn the self-healing techniques below, know that with time and practice, you are also likely to create your own set of techniques that work best for you.

These traditional positions are the same as the self-healing positions, only with the addition of three positions to help bring healing to your clients' legs and feet as well.

If you client is uncomfortable with light touch, you can also hover your hands over their body in the same positions. Please communicate with your client to ensure they have the most comfortable Reiki experience possible.

First Position – Palms Over Each Eye

In this position, you place the palms of your hands over each eye. This position allows for healing of the eyes, sinuses, brain, pituitary gland, pineal gland and the third eye chakra. This is the position used for eye strain, eye stress, headaches, migraines, anxiety, stress, fevers, allergies, colds and flus. Be sure to be gentle with your hands and do not squeeze the nose or apply too much pressure to their face.

Second Position – Palms on Each Side of the Face, Near Temples

In this position, you will gently place both of your palms on either side of your clients' face, right at the temples and/or over their ears. This position allows for continued healing of the eyes, sinuses, brain, pituitary gland, pineal gland and the third eye chakra; and, also provides healing to the ears as well. This is the position used for eye strain, eye stress, headaches, migraines, anxiety, stress, ear infections, hearing impairments, fevers, allergies, colds and flus.

Third Position – Hands Cradling Under the Head

In this position, your hands will cradle your client's head: place both palms directly underneath their head so that your fingertips are gentle holding their neck. You can access this by gently rocking their head to one side and slipping your hands under their head. Many clients fall asleep immediately when reiki is transmitted here, as this is the part of the body associated with sleep and deep rest.

Fourth Position- Palms on Each Side of the Neck

In this position, you place each of your palms on either side of their neck, just slightly underneath the ears. This position allows you to bring healing to their lungs, esophagus, pulmonary arteries, lymph nodes, vocal chords, thyroid, and the throat chakra. This is the position associated with healing lymphatic and thyroid disorders, artery and heart issues, asthma, laryngitis, fear of public speaking, and ensuring that their communications are clear and well heard.

Fifth Position – Palms Over the Sternum / Breastbone (Just Below Collarbone)

This position focuses on bringing healing to the upper lungs, heart, thymus gland (which is the gland responsible for stress), breasts, and the heart chakra. This is the position used to healing and treating asthma, breathing issues, pneumonia, heart issues and disease, breast cancer, chronic stress and/or anxiety, and matters related to relationships, self-love, love, and passion.

Sixth Position – Palms Over the Chest (Between Collarbone and Bellybutton)

In this position, you place their palms directly over their heart and chest area. This position brings continued healing to the same areas described in the third position.

Seventh Position – Palms Over the Belly Button

In this position, you place both of your palms directly over the bellybutton. This position brings healing to the stomach, pancreas, kidneys, gallbladder, liver, and is associated with the solar plexus chakra. This is the position to use when you are treating any health issues related to the digestive tract, liver, and kidneys. Additionally, since the solar plexus chakra is associated with creativity, this is a good position to work with if you are experiencing any blockages or lack of inspiration.

Eighth Position – Palms Under the Belly Button, Above the Groin

In this position, you need to place the palms of your hand just above their groin, but slightly below the bellybutton. This allows you to bring Reiki healing to the small intestines, large intestines, and colon. These positions not only bring additional healing for the digestive track, but also support with healing needs for anyone afflicted with celiac or irritable bowel syndrome.

Ninth Position – Palms On the Groin Area

In this position, you are to place the palms of their hands on either side of their groin. This position brings additional healing to the digestive and urinary systems and also heals any issues related to the reproductive organs, hormones, and pregnancy. This area of the body is also associated with the root chakra, so this healing position is also helpful for healing matters associated with security, safety, and financial opportunities.

Tenth Position – Palms on Each Leg

In this final position, you place both of your hands on either of their legs, and then slowly work the Reiki energy down to the soles of the feet. Some practitioners like to give a gentle tug on the heels of the feet so that they finish the Reiki healing session with a little bit of grounding energy work so that their clients can leave the session feeling strong and taller than ever.

Repeating the Reiki Healing on Both Sides

Some practitioners believe that Reiki healing needs to take place on both sides of the body, others believe that one side is just enough. If you feel that your client requires intensive healing due to intense emotional or physical distress, it is recommended that you repeat all of these same hand positions on the other side of the body. If your client is laying down, gently inform them after you are done with the feet that they will need to roll over so that you can work on the other side of the body.

Starting Out: Tips for Securing Reiki Clients

If you are unable to get clients right away for their healing practice, not to worry. Many healing and wellness centers offer group or community reiki opportunities. This allows you to give Reiki with other Reiki practitioners in a group setting. It is a great way to meet new people who, if they like your healing style, can become your future client.

Chapter 13: Level II Self Healing Techniques

The difference between a Level I and II self-healing practice is that with Level II, you are able to use and invoke the three symbols (Choku-Rei, Sei Hei Ki, and the Distance symbol) in your self-healing practice. You are welcome to incorporate these symbols with either the traditional Level I Usui hand positions we outlined in the Level I Self-Healing techniques chapter or you are welcome to incorporate these symbols into your own hand positions and techniques that work best for you.

Choose Your Intention

Since you are able to use the three different symbols, you are able to access a deeper form of Reiki healing that is not limited to the present moment. Focus on what your intentions for your self-healing practice are. Do you wish to simply enhance the strength of your regular, Level I based practice? If so, invoking the choku-rei symbol over each respective area of your body would work well. If you are interested in or are in need of healing a particular emotional challenge or would like to send healing energy to the past, present, or future moment that may even be the source of this distress, it would be good to incorporate the Sei Hei Ki and Distance Healing symbols with your practice.

Chapter 14 : Level II Healing Techniques for Others

Typically a Level II healing session with your client requires a lot of attention and effort on emotional healing, intensive physical healing through the use of the Choku Rei symbol, and, providing distance healing if your client is either unable to be physically present or requests that Reiki is sent to heal a past, present, or future issue.

Just because you are a Level II practitioner doesn't mean you are limited to working exclusively with symbols. In fact, these Level II techniques can be combined with the fundamental healing positions and techniques from Level I. The Level II symbols simply amplify the emotional and spiritual healing taking place and can enable you to work with your client remotely.

Choku Rei: The Power Symbol

Choku Rei is used to bring a significant amount of Reiki to the area that the symbol is drawn over. Choku Rei is especially helpful and effective when used over physical areas with chronic health issues, surgeries, injuries, or terminal illnesses.

Sei Hei Ki: The Emotional Healing Symbol

The healing process must also take place at the emotional level. Although some clients have emotional reactions to Reiki healing, it does not mean that they are emotionally healed. There are several strong theories in the medical and alternative medicine fields that suggest that one's emotional state can drastically affect one's physical wellbeing. That said, it is very important to also include the use of the Sei Hei Ki symbol in working with your client. If you client complains of a chronic health issue that doesn't seem to resolve no matter how many methods they use, consider using the Sei Hei Ki symbol in addition to your healing hand position. If you want up the ante on the efficacy of this work, you can draw the Choku Rei symbol before and after the Sei Hei Ki symbol. This technique is considered a powerful "Reiki sandwhich" since the Choku Rei symbol amplifies the power of the emotional healing symbol and process. If you do use this symbol, let your client know and prepare them to drink more water, caution them that some repressed memories may surface, and, ensure that they give themselves a little longer to heal after the session than usual.

Distance Healing Techniques

If your client is unable to be physically present, the distance symbol is just as good as healing them in person. Here are some traditional distance healing techniques that work well in lieu of an in-person healing session:

>The Surrogate
>
>You can use anything (such as a doll, toy, or even yourself) as a surrogate to channel Reiki. The most important thing you must do before you get started is that in your preparation to call Reiki to your hands, make sure that you clearly ask and let Reiki know that your surrogate is taking the place of whoever you are healing. A photograph, cushions, dolls, teddy bears, pens, crystals or the details of the person or thing

written on a piece of paper are all good examples of a surrogate. Heal the surrogate using the same hand positions as you would if they were in-person. Although in some cases you may need to use your imagination a bit, be sure that you pay extra attention to bring healing to the client's specific requests, even if it seems a bit silly to be doing so on an object that barely resembles a human being. In order to bring your utmost concentration to this task using this technique, I recommend that you do this one in the private comfort of where you practice self-Reiki so that you are not distracted by judgement or confusion that other people may have around you.

The Thigh and Knee Technique

This method will only require about 15 minutes of healing time and will require you to be seated. Once you're seated, make sure that your right knee and thigh the surrogate for the head and front of your client. Your right knee is your client head, your right mid thigh is your clients' body and the rest of your right thigh is your clients' legs and feet. The left knee and thigh represents the back of your clients head and body. Your left knee is the back of your clients head, your left mid thigh is your clients back and the rest of your left thigh represents the back of your clients' legs and feet. Using this model, you can easily conduct the motions of the healing techniques. This is a really easy to use, less complicated and significantly more discreet way of conducting a distance healing session on someone else.

Chapter 15 - Healing Relationships

While society teaches us that relationships are meant to lull us into a state of blissful ignorance, this is far from the truth. In reality, relationships are the laboratories in which every ounce of our own darkness and that of the other must be tested and transformed.

You only have to look back at your own life to realize that our hardest relationships are always with those whom we love most. Have you ever wondered why is this the case? Shouldn't these relationships be easy and blessed with perfect mutual understanding? Well, these relationships challenge us to the core because there is an important lesson for us to learn through every single one of our intimate connections. However, no matter what the curriculum might look like on the surface, the ultimate lesson is always the same: to forgive and to love unconditionally. Again, Reiki can help in creating beautiful relationships by transforming problems and negativity through the healing vibrations of the Universe.

Use the same techniques of distance healing as you would for a relationship. Draw and invoke Cho Ku Rei in both of your hands, then use the distance symbol and lovingly guide your hands or talk aloud to yourself about the emotional issues you would like for Reiki to heal during this session. Be gentle to yourself and take as long as you need with this type of work. Reiki is equally transformative to healing relationships as with the body, so be mindful of the fact and possibility that some relationships might need to be on the brink of ending in order for them to become stronger.

Reiki Relationship Healing Meditation

- Sit down in a comfortable position keeping your back straight.
- Take a few deep breaths allowing your body to relax completely.
- Bring your palms together in the Gassho position and set the intention to become a pure channel for Reiki energy to flow through you.
- Keep your eyes closed and feel the Reiki energy entering you through the crown chakra touching every part of your body.
- Focus your internal gaze in-between your eyebrows where the third eye is located.
- In your third eye, see this person with whom you have a problematic relationship.
- Now, write down the Reiki symbols covering their entire body.
- Visualize yourself in front of them and write down the Reiki symbols covering your entire body.
- Now, go ahead and hug this person. Say whatever loving words you would like to say to them. Witness how their feelings are transforming.
- In your third eye, retain the ideal vision that you have for this relationship. Watch yourself living in harmony with this person while both your hearts are radiating with the purest light of the Universe. Notice how this picture is contained within a globe of beautiful pink light.
- Write down the Reiki symbols on top of a harmonious picture of your togetherness. For instance, write down the Reiki symbols over a mental picture of the two of you holding each other in a tight embrace.

- Keep your focus on this mental picture while continuing to write down the Reiki symbols on it several times. Follow your inner guidance to know when you are ready to come out of the meditation.

- When you are ready to open your eyes slowly move your palms and fingers, rub your palms together and place them on your eyes. Gently open your eyes.

- Do this meditation every day without fail. There is no restriction on how many times you can do it. Do it whenever it feels right and good to your heart.

IMPORTANT NOTE: It will take some time for the healing of the relationship to take place. You must continue to believe that you have a beautiful relationship with the person in question even if their current actions are antithetical to this idea. Trust that your relationship has already transformed and that the only thing which exists between this person and you is pure love.

Another important thing to remember here is that sometimes healing of a relationship might bring about a completely unexpected result. For instance, the person might choose to walk away or the relationship might come to an abrupt end. Trust that everything is happening for everyone's highest good. Healing happens the very moment we ask for it, no matter what the outcome might be at the gross physical level.

Chapter 16 - Transforming Negative Situations and Problems

No matter how hopeless a problem or situation seems, it is never too late for Reiki to create miracles. Believe in miracles and you will experience them.

Here's how to go about transforming any difficult situation or major/minor life issue:

- Sit down in a comfortable position keeping your back straight.
- Take a few deep breaths allowing your body to relax completely.
- Bring your palms together in the Gassho position and set the intention to become a pure channel for Reiki energy to flow through you.
- Keep your eyes closed and feel the Reiki energy entering you through the crown chakra touching every part of your body.
- Focus your internal gaze in-between your eyebrows where the third eye is located.
- In your third eye center, visualize a blackboard. On this blackboard, you can see the problem or issue you have. Allow yourself to feel all the emotions that are coming up.
- Now, take an eraser and wipe off the entire picture. Watch how a new picture has taken over the place of the old one. In this new picture, everything is positive, joyous and harmonious. There is a bright glowing purple light surrounding this picture.

- Write down the Reiki symbols on top of this picture several times.

- From this moment on, retain this picture in your mind and never let the previous vision of the problem emerge again. Every time you find yourself worrying or being anxious, bring your awareness to this new picture and write down the Reiki symbols on it.

- Follow your inner guidance to know when you are ready to come out of the meditation. When you are ready to open your eyes slowly move your palms and fingers, rub your palms together and place them on your eyes. Gently open your eyes.

- Practice this meditation every day without fail until the situation has transformed completely, which it definitely would. However, you must remain detached from the outcome and not question when and how it is going to happen. You have to trust that the transformation has already taken place. Very soon you will find out that you are indeed right.

Chapter 17 - Aura Cleansing Exercises

Your aura is the unique magnetic field surrounding your physical body. Every person and every living thing has an aura. The size of one's aura depends upon the level of one's spiritual growth. A fearful and negative person's aura might be only a few inches wide while a spiritual master's aura can expand up to several kilometers.

Every thought we have affects our aura in either a positive way or a negative way. Clairvoyant individuals can clearly see the changes in people's aura as the person shifts from positive thoughts to negative or vice versa.

Protecting our aura from negativity and keeping is clean at all times is necessary for spiritual hygiene. If your aura is clean and relatively free of negativity, you will feel energetic and happy. Other people will be drawn to your positivity and you will attract more positive experiences into your life.

You must perform this aura cleansing exercise every morning and evening before starting your Reiki healing sessions and other meditation practices. Here's how to go about it:

- Sit down in a comfortable position while keeping your back straight.

- Take a few deep breaths and allow your body to relax completely.

- Imagine a globe of bright white light 6" above your head. Experience how this light is descending down and surrounding your entire body.

- Now, imagine a large golden comb with huge bristles 6" above your head. Visualize an invisible hand combing your aura from top to bottom. With each brush stroke, all the negativity is falling down into the earth where it will be transformed into pure white light.

- Continue combing your aura until you intuitively know that it is clean and free of all negativity.

- Now, visualize a golden pyramid surrounding your body and set the intention that from this moment on, only pure positive energy can touch you. If any negative energy or experience comes close to your aura they will only be able to touch the outer walls of this enormous golden pyramid which would then reflect it back to the Universe so that the energy can transform into the purest light of the Universe and return as a blessing to the sender. Remember, the more you bless the world, the more blessings you will experience in your own life.

- Perform this aura cleansing exercise as a precursor to the rest of your practice. Think of this as being similar to the act of taking a shower before getting dressed for the day.

Chapter 18 - How to Increase Your Life Force Energy

Every living thing has life force energy. The more life force energy one has, the healthier and happier one is. Have you noticed how some people seem to be extremely attractive even if they might not be conventionally beautiful? This is again because of a higher amount of life force energy. Similarly, people who are negative or those who constantly criticize and talk ill of others have a repulsive aura. We don't enjoy being in their presence even if they aren't even saying anything at all in the moment. Remember, everything in the Universe is energy and energy never stops communicating.

Take these steps to increase your life force energy. Not only will you experience a positive change in yourself but your life will also transform from the inside-out:

- Maintain a clean vegetarian diet (of possible) and stay away from intoxicants including alcohol and cigarettes as much as possible.
- Eat lots of raw or lightly cooked organic vegetables.
- Incorporate plenty of fresh organic fruits into your diet.
- Bless everyone you meet. Every time you bless someone else, the Universe is bringing those blessings back to you manyfold.
- Treat everyone with love and compassion. Practice unconditional love towards every creature. Nothing increases life force energy as profoundly as practicing unconditional love. This kind of love has the power to heal any disease and miraculously transform any situation.
- Refrain from anger as anger can rapidly deplete life-force energy. This holds true for all negative emotions. Every time

you feel angry or negative, bless the person or situation and send unconditional love to it.

- Remain pure in your intentions and speak from your heart. If you are saying something while feeling something else in your heart, your words and actions are not pure. Ensure that there your inner feelings and outer words/actions are in sync at all times.

- Always remain honest and act with integrity. Dishonesty stems from a place of fear and fear can rapidly deplete your aura of life force energy.

While these steps sound simple, if practiced with sincerity, they will completely change your life. Your face will radiate with an extraordinary inner glow that others will find mystifying and yet, at the same time, irresistibly attractive.

Chapter 19 - Using the Power of Reiki to Attract anything you want

Reiki is a powerful tool to assist with manifestation. However, before starting your practice, you must write down on paper exactly what you want. You must write your desires as if they have already happened in the present. For example, instead of saying, "I will work at a wonderful and rewarding job," you can say, "I am working at a wonderful and rewarding job." Also, be as specific as possible. For instance, don't say, I want to have a lot of money, instead, specify exactly how much money is enough for you and write your desire down as if you have already received this amount.

One important rule here is to never write the name of a specific person with whom you desire a relationship or a specific company where you want to work. Always write down the qualities you would like your partner to have or the qualities you would like your ideal company to have.

- Write down your goals with so much precision that you can form a mental picture of them.

- At the end of your spiritual practice or meditation session, bring this picture up and watch it unfolding with precision in your mind's eye.

- Imagine a golden globe of light descending and surrounding this picture.

- Write down the Reiki symbols on this ideal picture of your goals and enjoy feeling all the good emotions that you are already experiencing.

- Retain this happy and positive feeling as this will make you a vibrational match for your heart's desire. Don't doubt or slip into negativity as this will negatively impact the vibrational harmony you have managed to achieve through this practice.

- Every time you think about you goal, visualize this ideal picture within a golden globe of light. Emotions are your power here, so allow yourself to keep feeling good at all times.

Chapter 20 - The Importance of Diet and Exercise

Maintaining a clean diet and a regular exercise regimen is pivotal to any spiritual practice as they purify the body and mind making it more receptive to the higher vibrations of the Universe. Below are some simple diet and exercise tips to incorporate with your regular Reiki practice:

- Eat a clean vegetarian diet. Even if you can't totally give up on meat, increase the quantity of vegetarian food you include in your diet.
- Drink plenty of water throughout the day. Stay away from refrigerated water as it is not good for digestion. Instead, develop a habit of drinking lukewarm water or water at room temperature.
- Try eating fresh home-cooked meals as much as possible. Cook every meal with love and happiness. If you have received the level 2 initiation, then you can also mentally write the Reiki symbols on the food that you are cooking. This will further enhance the life force energy of the meal. Any person eating that meal will not only receive the nutrition of the meal but that person will also absorb the healing energy of Reiki.
- Stay away from processed packaged food.
- Don't consume food items with chemicals, colors and additives.
- Start your day with a tablespoon of apple cider vinegar in warm water.
- Practice yoga and pranayama if you can.
- Engage in some kind of vigorous exercise that makes your body sweat (for at least, 20 minutes every day).

- Avoid eating right before your Reiki and meditation practice. If you must, then make sure you are eating something light and easy to digest.
- Reduce your intake of sugar and salt.
- Maintain a regular schedule for eating, sleeping and waking up. Stick to this schedule even on weekends.
- Take regular walks in nature.
- Laughter is a wonderful exercise for the mind and the soul. Therefore, laugh as much as possible.

Chapter 21: Meditation for Exploring Your Connection to Reiki

Let's focus on how your relationship with Reiki can grow over time by first exploring your relationship to Reiki. In this session, you might want to read aloud the following script and record your own voice reading these instructions aloud so you can play it back and work on your relationship to Reiki in order toe be a stronger healer. Please find a quiet and comfortable space to sit, relax, and tune into yourself:

Exploring Your Connection to Reiki Script

- Inhale deeply and close your eyes, slowly feeling the world around you fade away. Slowly breathe in and out, relaxing your neck and shoulders, breathing deeply and loosening your arms, hands, lower back, ankles and feet to relax. Take a few slow, deep breaths, gently easing yourself into a calm and peaceful state.

- Observe how you feel right now, physically and emotionally. Do you feel balanced, a little off balanced, or not your usual self? As you continue to take slow, steady breaths, keeping your eyes closed and body relaxed, notice how your body and your mind tell you how you are feeling right now. What do you need to feel completely well and good? As an emerging healer, how would you heal yourself right now? Take a few moments to visualize how you would heal yourself -- what would you do? Feel? Wear? How would you know you were completely healed - what emotions, feelings, sensations, and thoughts would you have? Take some time now to visualize how you would heal yourself and what that would feel like.

- Now let's think about your connection to healing and your desire to work with Reiki. What are your experiences with healing and Reiki? What about these experiences appeals to your goals, and, how will you use these healing sessions? Take a few moments to think about some goals for your healing journey now - including any answers you are hoping to find about how Reiki can support you.

- When you are ready, slowly open your eyes and bring your awareness back into the room. You may want to use this time to record some of your observations and goals for healing. If you are not sure what you are hoping to achieve with Reiki or your healing journey, try listening to this session a few times - allow your gut instinct to guide you. Our understanding of our intentions is essential for working with Reiki: the clearer the goal, the more you can focus your healing energy on achieving it. Over time, you may also find that your healing goals change as you develop your healing practice. Trust that you know what you need, even if it might not seem obvious yet. This is the first step on your healing journey.

Reiki for Emotional Well Being

- At the disadvantage of the Level I practitioner, many of the emotional healing techniques are for Level II practitioners only, typically because they receive special symbols in their attunement process that allow them to specifically target emotionally-caused ailments.

- In light of this challenge, below is an incredible meditation that can be used as a nice alternative (or supplement, if you are a Level II practitioner) for emotional healing. Enjoy.

Emotional Well Being Reiki Healing Techniques

- lose your eyes and inhale deeply, and exhale deeply. Call Reiki into the palms of your hands.

- First, you will be healing the areas of your head that are associated with stress, emotional overwhelm, cognitive impairments and anxiety. Slowly bring your hands over the top of your head, hovering them about an inch from the top of your forehead, and concentrate on the flow of Reiki, visualizing and guiding Reiki with your hands in a slow, steady stream around your head, beginning with your forehead, working up to the top of your head, hovering to the back of your head near the base of your neck.

- Slowly work your hands from the back of the neck all the way to your forehead again, focusing on the flow of Reiki moving throughout your head. Bring your hands to rest on top of your head, with your palms on either side of your head, fingers facing toward the back of your head and your palms closest to your forehead. Focus on the flow of Reiki here.

- The top of the head stores a lot of mental energy, worry, fear, and emotional and cognitive processing; so, if these are issues you are particularly looking to heal, give them special attention by placing your hands here as long as you need to. Observe any imagery, sensations and images that may come up for you in this spot.

- When you are ready, keep one hand on the top of your forehead and place your other hand just behind your head, above the base of your neck. This position helps to balance displaced energy from headaches and mental exhaustion, balancing the energies to your whole head to be processed and cleared, which helps to ground you.

- If worry, doubt, emotional confusion or tension headaches are also troubling you, guide your hands to hover just above the space in-between your eyebrows, concentrating on the flow of Reiki over this region, which is often referred to as the "third eye". Here, our emotions tend to get trapped and tangled up when we cannot immediately release them. Hover your hands gently over this spot, making small circles with your hands, observing how this feels for you.

- If you are experiencing a lot of eye strain, blurred vision, emotional fatigue, allergies, or emotional tension (such as not being able to cry to release what you are feeling), place the palms of your hands over your eyes and visualize Reiki wash over your eyelids, alleviating the pressure on either side and behind your eyes.

- If you feel that you are receiving and hearing a lot of emotional or stressful information that you do not want to process or think about, your ears, believe it or not, will keep this energy stuck.

- If you feel that you "don't want to hear" about a situation anymore, you should routinely heal your ears by placing your hands over your ears, using Reiki to wash through your ears, and ask Reiki to help clear the unnecessary noise and help you hear the pure truth surrounding you so that you feel less overwhelmed.

- Emotional and stressful tensions can unconsciously make us clench our jaws or grind our teeth in our sleep as a means of release. To help move this energy along, place your hands on either side of your jaw, with your fingertips resting just under your ears and have Reiki flow from your hands up either sides of your jaw. You may wish to release your hands from your jaw and have them over your jaw and guide them up to your temples and back down, depending on how severe you tense your jaw.

- After trying any or all of the above techniques, end your healing session by creating a protective and healing shield around your head and neck, visualizing and affirming to yourself that you will be more balanced experiencing and releasing emotions. To do this, keep your hands charged with Reiki and hover your hands under your chin, with your pinkies touching each other. Visualize a warm shield of light branching out from your hands to connect and meet at the top of your head, this warm light feeling like a soft and safe place. Keep your hands here as long as you need to.

- Close your connection to Reiki when you feel you are ready to move on. This is also an excellent technique to maintain a peaceful and calm state, especially if you are about to do something stressful or emotionally challenging. For example, try using this technique daily right before you are about to work or have a hard conversation with someone.

- The more you use these techniques to intercept the onset of headaches, migraines, and emotional or mental imbalances, the less frequent their symptoms will be, and you may find that your symptoms will be less intense or gradually disappear.

- You may find that one particular hand position or technique works better for you than others. Experiment and see what works best for you. You can also try combining all of these techniques into one longer session that focuses on maintaining and restoring balance to all of these emotional and cognitive centers. See what works for you.

Reiki for Environmental Relationships and Healing

The following are some powerful techniques that will help you to scan your energetic field, also known as your aura, which is an extension of your body's internal energies. Your aura is influenced by your energies and the energies of your environment (including people, places, and things). The skills you'll learn in this session will help you develop an awareness of how your body and your environment contribute to your aura's state, and how your aura reciprocates these energies back into your body and environment.

You may want to consider reading the below directions out loud and creating a recording of yourself, so that you can repeat this exercise as many times as you'd like with ease:

Close your eyes and slowly breathe in and out, softening your neck, your shoulders, breathing deeply and relaxing your arms, hands, lower back, ankles and feet. Take slow, deep breathes as you gently feel yourself relaxing and easing into a calm and peaceful state.

When you are ready, invoke Reiki into your hands, using your preferred method of calling in Reiki. Feel Reiki's powerful and bright healing light emerge into your palms. When you feel that Reiki is very charged in your palms, slowly raise your hands, making sure that your palms are facing outward from your body. Slowly open your eyes and visualize Reiki as two bright balls in your hands, churning around like two spinning spheres, as your hands slowly first fall to your lap and then make their way up through to your head, hovering above your body. What do you feel or see around you? Slowly keep your palms guiding up to your head, then slowly move them back down and around your body, imagining the spheres of Reiki in your palms scanning this field around your body several times.

This is your aura, your energetic field. Notice what it feels like: is it buzzing, flowing, soft, or hard? Does it buzz or vibrate as you move around it, or is it stable and firm? Do you visualize colors as you move your hands around your body? Is it warm or cool? Breathing deeply, keep moving your hands around your energy field and observe its unique qualities. If you would like to grow your awareness of your aura, try this exercise when you are experiencing different emotions such as joy, sadness, anxiety, and anger. Notice how shifts in your emotional state affect your energetic field.

Now, we will use this technique to explore the energy around you. Slowly open your eyes and keep your palms extended from your body in front of you. Keep the flow of the bright spheres of Reiki strong in your palms. You will now begin to scan your environment and feel its energies. Slowly extend your arms and palms as far as possible. Imagine you are shooting a beam of light that boomerangs all around the space around you, and, when it returns to your palms, brings back the energies, feelings, sights, and sounds of your environment to your hands. What do you feel back from the space around you? How does the energy that was transmitted back to you tell this to you? Try sending Reiki energy out into the environment around you and receiving it back a few times, observing any differences and subtleties. Know that when you feel these energies, you are safe.

Reiki, as universal life energy, does not allow for the adsorption or depletion of energy: it simply connects us with energy so that we may harmonize it.

Another technique you may use to explore the energies of your environment is to focus your attention back on those balls of Reiki energy in your palms and hover your palms close to the walls, desks, doorways, chairs, and frequently used or trafficked areas, feeling how these areas may have energies radiating off of them that your palms detect. This is similar to how you detected your aura's properties earlier in this session. If you are outdoors, you can use this same technique with nature, feeling the plants, water, earth, and wind around you. What do these places and things feel like in your hands without touching them? What colors, textures, shapes, or temperatures do you feel?

Play around with this a little bit and record your findings over time. You will find that you will develop your own way of observing common themes, for example, a doorway may feel like it is empty and buzzing with the remnants of all the activity from people who have passed in and out of it.

As you finish exploring the energetic fields of yourself and your environment, bring your palms back together, clasping them firmly and close your connection to Reiki in the way that you prefer to do so. Thank Reiki for guiding you safely to explore your energy and the energy around you.

Take a moment to record some of your thoughts and observations. Doing this exercise regularly will help you explore the many unique energetic properties we and our environments are composed of, which will continue to build your understanding of working with diverse energies using Reiki.

Chapter 22 - Reiki for Animals, Children and the Elderly

Reiki can be used on every living thing for healing, personal development, deep relaxation and stress relief. The many benefits we receive from Reiki, giving or receiving, are meant to be shared and experienced with all beings. Animals, children and the elderly are incredibly receptive to Reiki Energy. Providing reiki to these three different audiences is gaining a lot of popularity lately, mostly because it is extremely rewarding. Children, the elderly, and animals are very appreciative and respond joyfully to receiving Reiki, which makes it a wonderful experience for both the healer and the receiver! Reiki is a very effective therapy for these populations, which is why it may be so incredibly rewarding for the practitioner.

If you are just beginning your healing practice, many hospitals, elder care homes and centers, and veterinarian clinics are offering Reiki! Since this is an emerging trend in holistic health, this is an excellent opportunity for you to introduce a powerful, transformative and loving experience to a warm, receptive, and curious population that will appreciate your nurturing healing.

Special Instructions for Preparing Animals and Babies for Reiki

Animals and babies need to be sitting or resting on your lap in order for a Reiki healing to successfully take place. Animals and babies are highly sensitive to Reiki and immediately respond to it. Just like adult humans, animals and babies are also able to feel a lot better and can recover from illness, disease, and emotional pain from neglect, fear, or even abuse.

The Reiki healing hand positions are the same for babies and animals. Since these populations are prone to shifting and moving around a lot, prepared to be creative! It's ok if you can't get the exact same hand positions with these populations – it's the effort for giving reiki in a safe, fun, and relaxed matter that counts the most. Pay attention to their body language, especially since babies and animals can't talk to let you know how they are feeling – instead, they will be sure to show it!

If, for some reason, any of these populations are uncomfortable receiving hands-on Reiki treatment, you can also choose to heal them using distant healing techniques, even if they are in the same room. That way, you can safely and comfortably send them Reiki without having to be directly on them.

Reiki and Animals, Children and the Elderly

Reiki works really well for this population in the following instances:

• When they are just born

• When they are ill: Reiki helps the healing process and works with any type of medical or veterinary treatment.

• When they have been through a trauma: they can use loving energy after they've experienced any type of abuse, loss, or move, or if they seem to exhibit depression or other behavioural disorder. Even if you don't know what the problem is, you can use Reiki to help.

• Regularly, every day, to upkeep some balanced energy so that they do not become suscepitible to stress or illness.

• You can also Reiki their food, water, medication, doctor's visits for positive, balanced, and vital outcomes for their highest good.

Communicating with These Special Populations

Since animals, children and the elderly are so fragile, they can definitely respond differently to Reiki depending on their type of illness, personality, and how well they know and trust you. Here are some general characteristics to keep an eye out for so you can better understand their healing needs and to make sure that it is still ok to heal them throughout the Reiki session:

• A baby may begin to cry hysterically or an animal may bark, growl, screech, fly, hiss, buck or run away as a way of telling you it doesn't want to be touched. If this happens and you know the animal is sick or in pain and needs Reiki then you can still treat the animal by using distant Reiki.

• Although they might, at first, let you perform hands-on Reiki, after awhile they may want to shift positions or begin to look at you with skepticism or discomfort. If this happens, change to a distance Reiki treatment instead.

• Animals, especially if they are around self-healing Reiki sessions, may tell you it wants Reiki by coming near you when you are giving Reiki to yourself or someone else.

• If you at any time sense a change in the animal mood or energy and are concerned for your own safety, stop the treatment immediately and continue sending reiki from a safe distance.

Chapter 23 - Reiki and Other Healing Modalities

Reiki can complement and enhance the effectiveness of almost any other method of healing you may currently be working with or may work with in the future. Reiki energy balances the subtle frequencies of the person's energetic body as it is being received.

Reiki can be combined with any other medical, psychological, or alternative medicine therapy to achieve deeper and more profound healing. In Fact, Combining Healing Modalities can help to increase the benefits of a Reiki healing session for the recipient. Many hospitals, health clinics and psychiatric research centers across the United States are beginning to incorporate Reiki in their medical practice, especially with patients who are afflicted with life-threatening and incurable diseases.

Remember if you are going to combine healing modalities you must first explain to your client what you intend to do during the session and get permission from them to use more than just Reiki. You could of course just use Reiki and remain with the viewpoint that Reiki will go where it is needed and do what is needed to facilitate change and healing.

Chapter 24 – Reiki Healing Tools for Practitioners

If you are ready to take the next step in your Reiki healing practice, such as own your own professional healing service or center, you'll need to invest in a few affordable tools for the trade. Here is an essential toolkit of all the items you will need to start your professional practice and/or space:

Massage Table

This is the most essential tool – the table. Whether you are an emerging practitioner, Master, or a freshly graduated Level I student eager to start working with clients, the most essential tool for you to invest in for your Reiki practice is a comfortable, easy to use massage table. Since these tables are traditionally used for massage practices, their name appears very singular to that profession; however, all energy healing and Reiki practitioners use the same resources and tools because they are easy, affordable, and relatively effective for serving a client.

Since many clients feel extremely relaxed (and, sometimes even fall asleep during treatment), the Reiki table should be like a good mattress: strong, durable, soft, long-lasting, and easy on the wallet. Your client's physiological and psychological needs drive what type of table will be best for your private or community healing practice.

Additionally, your needs as Reiki practitioner also factor in to the type of features you want with your Reiki table. Since many practitioners provide healing in their homes, portable, easy to assemble tables are preferred for easy storage. You will also want to consider your own comfort as you administer Reiki, especially if you prefer to sit or stand.

Reiki tables borrow elements from massage tables; however, since Reiki does not involve physically aggressive bodywork, many features are overwhelming and unnecessary for consideration for Reiki, especially for those of you who are buying tools like this for the first time.

Since Reiki tables borrow elements from the massage and body work industry, there are several types of very important features available depending on you and your client's needs. Some tables are more adjustable, portable, and comfortable than others and of course, this will be contingent on the price and quality of materials used for their design. Depending on the size and scale of your practice and budget, each of these features will vary. Whether you are a first-time buyer or looking to invest in a more expensive model, these are the three main considerations for you to keep in mind when you are shopping around for a Reiki table:

Adjustable Height

As you will find during your career as a Reiki healer, not only will different techniques support each client differently, but you will also be at varying heights in relationship to your client. Reiki requires you to comfortably and fully extend both your hands and arms on and over your client. Depending on your client's height or your own preference for sitting or standing while you conduct the healing, you'll want to consider a table that is height adjustable. If you see multiple clients back to back, the option to adjust the table so that you can sit for a few sessions is a nice luxury for your own comfort for those super long hours. No one wants to keep shifting their weight as they are working on their client or feeling distracted by discomfort in not be able to fully reach your clients' head or back – your discomfort would be a noticeable distraction to your client so it is important to make sure that the massage table you are considering is adjustable.

Portable

Most tables are portable; however, you should find out just what it is about the tables that make them so portable. For example, some tables have additional knobs, springs, and aluminum features that allow them to be set up pretty fast. This efficiency, however, often times comes at the cost of having a much heavier table than you bargained for. If you are a home-based practitioner, you'll also want to consider a table that has built-in handles on the side, is lightweight, or comes with an easy to use carrying case so that you can easily store the table if you are using the same room in your home for various purposes.

Comfortable

Client comfort is an underestimated component for a wonderfully successful healing Reiki experience that will culminate in a huge return on investment for your business. Since your client is laying down on their stomach and back for at least 30 minutes, you will definitely want them to be as comfortable as possible. Consider the thickness, softness, durability, and firmness of each massage table. You'll want your client to feel like they are about to get the best sleep of their life or to feel as relaxed as possible, especially since they are receiving a treatment outside of their familiar day-to-day environments. A comfortable table is also very welcoming for first-timers to Reiki who might be tensed up and nervous and unsure of what to expect. Clients who have particular physical ailments or psychological needs would greatly benefit from feeing like they are comfortable, safe, and relaxed throughout the Reiki healing experience – you don't want them to feel like they are at just another doctor's office, that's for sure!

Sufficient Support for Heavier Weight

You will want to make sure that your new table will be able to withstand all of your client's needs, including making sure they are safe and firmly secure. It would be important to ensure that your table of choice doesn't shake, creak, or snap based on their weight. Depending on the tables' materials, some tables can handle heavier weight loads than others.

Face Cradle

The next essential item to include in your emerging Reiki practice toolbox is to invest in an equally durable, and high quality face cradle for your client's comfort. Clients will need to comfortably rest face down when they are on their stomachs and a pillow doesn't really do the job with comfort. Since most massage tables are universal in design, face cradles can easily fit and attach themselves to any table you end up buying. They are typically sold separately and are often forgotten about when it's time to make the investment.

Reiki Table Sheets

Since the table should be as comfortable as the bed of your client's dreams, you will also want to invest in some comfortable and easy to clean sheets for the table. You can't use regular bed sheets for clinical, healing use, so here are several essentials factors to consider when buying sheets for your Reiki table:

Factor 1 – Hypoallergenic

Your client may have incredibly sensitive skin or you may be in an environment where strong hygienic practices are absolutely imperative. That said, you want to make sure that your sheets are hypoallergenic. Hypoallergenic sheets prohibit dust mites, bacteria, hair, dead skin, and even sweat from literally destroying the fabric and transferring onto another person. Although these massage sheet fabrics may be a bit more expensive than the rest, you are investing in your client's safety and comfort.

Factor 2 – Oil-Resistant

Many Reiki healers like to use essential oils or massage grade oils (especially for those of you who like to integrate massage into your Reiki practice) when working with clients. Oils can actually be pretty penetrable and harsh on most fabrics, possibly ruining them forever. If you like to use essential oils, no matter the grade, make sure to read each product description carefully so that you purchase sheets that are oil-resistant.

Factor 3 – Breathable Fabric

Not all fabric blends are equal. Your client will want to get nice and relaxed and comfortable during their Reiki session. The last thing anyone wants to feel is overheated, itchy, and uncomfortable during a special experience that is supposed to help them feel better and relax. Even if your client loves heavy flannels, make sure that they aren't going to start sweating buckets the longer they are laying down, otherwise that completely defeats the purpose of relaxing, doesn't it?

Chapter 25 – Detecting and Healing Negative Energy: Techniques and Meditation

An energetic blockage feels like Reiki isn't flowing strongly throughout your hands or into your body when you are performing a healing session. Energetic blockages are the result of pent up emotions that were not released fully, unexpressed thoughts, opinions, needs, or wants, and also the absorption of negative energy, words, or emotions from someone that you have not processed or let go of. Blockages prevent us from feeling like we can move forward in our lives from particular situations, create new solutions and opportunities, or let go of things that are bothering us or no longer serving us. As a result, blockages make us feel helpless, which in turn, makes these blockages bigger and bigger over time.

Let's first begin by focusing our awareness into ourselves to detect where we may have energetic blockages. Take a few slow, deep breaths as you close your eyes, paying attention to how you feel right now. You may find that negative feelings first or more readily come to you as you reflect on your current state. Allow yourself to fully feel and experience these negative emotions and observe their impact on your body. Do you feel your body tensing up in certain areas? Do you feel numbness, aching, or pressure in other areas as you work through these emotions? Slowly guide your awareness to the places you feel your emotions are coming from: this is where an energetic blockage will be found.

Take a few steady breaths as you work through finding and visualizing each energetic blockage. Use your intuition to sense what the blockage looks like, what it feels like, and the energies surrounding the blockage. Breathe deeply as you do this and give yourself lots of time to freely process the emotions, memories, and sensations that may come up through this process. Once you feel you have fully identified the blockage, its source, and properties, you are ready to heal yourself from it.

Take a few deep breaths in and out, and invoke Reiki into your hands. Slowly guide your hands to each area where you identified an energetic blockage, keeping your breath slow and steady. Cup your hands around the blockage, and visualize and feel Reiki energy dissolving it slowly. As you do this, additional memories and feelings may resurface for you. Do you feel a tingling, buzzing, burning or extremely cold sensation? Pay attention to how your hands feel as you pass a significant amount of Reiki energy to dissolve this blockage. If you are concerned you have lost your connection to Reiki in this process because you no longer feel your hands warming up, this means that the blockage is deeply embedded.

Try hovering your hands over the blockage site, and visualize Reiki charging down on the area like a hurricane with bright flashes of lightning coming down and through your body, whipping energy around and throughout your blockages. Ask Reiki to dissolve and disintegrate all that is holding you back, that you no longer want to hold onto whatever is keeping you from owning your own power. As you focus your intentions on dissolving these blockages, affirm to yourself that you do not wish to hold onto these energies any longer.

It may take several sessions for a blockage to fully leave the body and you may feel different types of sensations as you work in these areas. Take a few moments now to breathe deeply and explore what is coming up for you as you continue to heal the blockage. Ask yourself why you are holding onto this blockage and why you are afraid to let go of it. While you are guiding Reiki to remove the blockage, affirm that you are ready for this blockage to leave and that you accept all responsibility to process the energies that come with allowing the blockage to be removed.

When you are done, bring your palms back together, clasping them firmly and thank Reiki for guiding you safely to explore your blockages and healing them for your highest good.

Energetic blockages are one of the most common negative energies you will detect in a Reiki session. Be sure to record some notes and observations on the properties of each of your blockages, observing their characteristics such as shape, color, texture, sound, and any imagery associated with these energies. Also observe the feeling in your palms - does Reiki feel like it barely flowing or was it flowing excessively? Over time, you will learn how your body is healing these blockages with Reiki by noticing consistent signals your body is communicating to you about blockages.

Additional Meditation and Healing Meditation: Chords

If, during an aura scan or self-healing session, you felt like something was piercing your energy, or, images of a particular situation or person's words or actions kept coming to the surface, you encountered a chord clinging to your energy.

Chords carry the influences and residues of emotionally impactful persons and their words, actions, and energies. Chords feel like thick ropes, thorns, beams, or swords that pierce our physical and emotional bodies. Since we have not let go of these actions or relationships, their negative residue pierces us over and over again each time we think about them or the situation.

Chords can be detected the same way you detected energetic blockages. First, begin by focusing your awareness into yourself. Take several deep, steady breaths and close your eyes. Pay attention to how you feel. As you have experienced with energetic blockages in our prior session, you may still find that negative feelings are more easily coming to you right now. Allow yourself to fully feel and experience these negative emotions and observe their impact on your body. Do you feel a sinking or stabbing sensation in your body when you work through these motions? Slowly guide your awareness to the places you feel your emotions are coming from: this is where a chord will be found.

Take a few steady breaths as you work through finding and visualizing each chord. Use your intuition to define the properties of your chords: what it feels like, and the energies surrounding the blockage. Breathe deeply as you do this and give yourself lots of time to freely process the emotions, memories, and sensations that may come up through this process. Once you feel you have a good grasp on the source and nature of your chords, you are ready to begin to heal them.

Take a few deep breaths in and out, and invoke Reiki into your hands. Slowly guide your hands to each area where you identified a chord. To heal a chord, they must be pulled out of your energy, much like a sword being pulled from a stone.

Guide your palms to "clasp" around the chord, imagining it as an actual physical manifestation that you must pull out. Ask Reiki for assistance and visualize its healing energy pushing the chord from inside the body as you also "pull" it out with your hands. Visualize your energy and Reiki energy pushing this unwanted relationship, situation, or its residue out of you, and ask that it never return. As you pull the chord out of you, affirm to yourself that you no longer need this negative influence in your life as it does not align itself for your highest good.

When you feel that you have pulled it out entirely, thrash it out of your hands and visualize it vanishing into the ether, evaporating into nothingness. Place your hands over the area from which you pulled this negative energy out and transmit Reiki for a prolonged time into it, asking that it heal any residual wounds from this chord. When you are done, bring your palms back together, clasping them firmly and thank Reiki for guiding you safely to explore your blockages and healing them for your highest good.

It may take several sessions for a chord to be fully pulled from the body; and, the deeper the chord, the more resistance and fear you may feel in releasing it because you have coped with it for so long. Take a few moments now to breathe deeply and explore what is coming up for you as you continue to free yourself from the chord. Ask yourself why you are holding onto this chord and why you are afraid to let go of it. While you are guiding Reiki to help pull out the chord, affirm that you are ready for this blockage to leave and that you accept all responsibility to process the energies that come with allowing the chord and its connections to be removed from you.

As always, be sure to record some notes and observations on the properties of each of your chords, observing their characteristics such as shape, color, texture, sound, and any imagery associated with these energies, especially the interpersonal relationship and the reasons why you may not have been willing to let go of their negative influences on you. Blockages and chords are best treated through regular self-healing sessions.

Conclusion - Tips to Maintain a Daily Practice

- Set aside a particular time for your practice and do it every day at the same without fail.

- In order to make yourself more relaxed, you can light a candle and/or incense before starting the practice.

- You can have some kind of soft soothing music playing in the background. The sound of a waterfall can be especially relaxing.

- You can create a special meditation room or even a meditation corner. This space can have objects that you hold sacred.

- Creating a meditation altar with symbolic sacred objects is also a great idea.

- Set your goal as doing the practice for 21 days without any break. Repeat this at the end of every 21 days.

- You can maintain a journal writing down how long you practiced, what all you did, the changes you are experiencing, your goals, etc. This is excellent for keeping track of your progress and to keep yourself accountable.

- Don't lose heart when problems come up. Instead, increase the amount of effort you are putting into your practice.

Remember, consistency is the key here. Little by little, your life is guaranteed to change. Just stay on the path and NEVER GIVE UP!

Printed in Great Britain
by Amazon